ON LINE

Miracle
T·O·U·C·H

*A Complete Guide to Hands-On Therapies
That Have the Amazing Ability to Heal*

DEBRA FULGHUM BRUCE
FOREWORD by Dolores Krieger, Ph.D., RN

Miracle
T·O·U·C·H

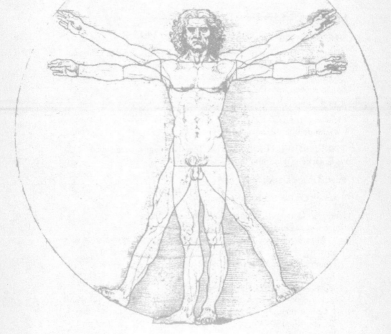

THREE RIVERS PRESS · NEW YORK

Note to Readers:
The material in this book is for information purposes only. It is not intended to serve as a diagnosis tool or prescription manual, or to replace the advice and care of your medical doctor. Although every effort has been made to provide the most up-to-date information about healing touch and other alternative therapies, the information in this field is rapidly changing. Therefore, we strongly recommend that you consult with your doctor before attempting any of the treatments or programs discussed in this book.

To protect their privacy, pseudonyms have been used for the individual patients and case stories mentioned in this book.

Copyright © 2003 by Debra Fulghum Bruce

Foreword copyright © 2003 by Dolores Krieger, Ph.D., RN

Published by Three Rivers Press, New York, New York.
Member of the Crown Publishing Group, a division of Random House, Inc.
www.randomhouse.com

THREE RIVERS PRESS and the Tugboat design are registered trademarks of Random House, Inc.

Printed in the United States of America

DESIGN BY ELINA D. NUDELMAN

Library of Congress Cataloging-in-Publication Data
Bruce, Debra Fulghum, 1951–
    Miracle touch : a complete guide to hands-on therapies that have the
  amazing ability to heal / by Debra Fulghum Bruce, foreword by
  Dolores Krieger.—1st ed.
      p.   cm.
    Includes bibliographical references.
    1. Touch—Therapeutic use.   2. Alternative medicine.   [DNLM:
  1. Complementary Therapies—Popular Works.   2. Therapeutic
  Touch—Popular Works.   WB 890 B8855m 2003]   I. Krieger,
  Dolores.   II. Title.
  RZ999 .B676   2003
  615.5—dc21   2002007443

ISBN 0-609-80734-X

10 9 8 7 6 5 4 3 2 1

First Edition

To Zoe Emmanuelle Bockenek

A precious gift from God whose presence has touched our lives

Born May 5, 2001

Acknowledgments

We have received generous assistance, along with a wealth of revealing testimonies, from a very select group of professionals. We express our gratitude to the following:

HARRIS H. MCILWAIN, M.D., author of *The Fibromyalgia Handbook* (Holt, 1999) and *The Super Aspirin Cure for Arthritis* (Bantam, 1999) and rheumatologist and geriatric specialist with Tampa Medical Group, P.A., Tampa, Florida.

KIMBERLY MCILWAIN, M.D., Tampa, Florida.

DR. GEORGE PRATT AND DR. PETER T. LAMBROU, authors of *Instant Emotional Healing: Acupressure for the Emotions* (Broadway Books, 2000) and codevelopers of Emotional Self-Management. Pratt and Lambrou are on staff at Scripps Memorial Hospital, La Jolla, California, and on the faculty of the University of California at San Diego.

DR. WILLIAM SEARS, author of *The Baby Book* and *The Pregnancy Book* (Little, Brown, 1993 and 1997), professor of pediatrics at University of California, Irvine, and pediatrician in San Clemente, California.

SAM THATCHER, M.D., PH.D., author of *Making a Baby* (Ballantine, 2000) and *Poly Cystic Ovary Syndrome* (Perspectives Press, 2000) and obstetrician/gynecologist and reproductive endocrinologist, Center for Applied Reproductive Science, Johnson City, Tennessee.

JOEL C. SILVERFIELD, M.D., rheumatologist with Tampa Medical Group, P.A., Tampa, Florida.

NURSE HEALERS PROFESSIONAL ASSOCIATES INTERNATIONAL, The Official Organization of Therapeutic Touch, Salt Lake City, Utah.

HEALING TOUCH INTERNATIONAL, Lakewood, Colorado.

THOMAS MARY D'ILLON WITH THE FLOWER ESSENCE SOCIETY, Nevada City, California.

CHERYL STROUP, Reiki master teacher and California-based author of *The Holy Art of Reiki* (Samuel Wesier, 2002).

MILLIE ANDERSON, therapeutic-touch practitioner, Manhattan Beach, California.

DEB WEST, M.S.W., Traverse City, Michigan.

RAYMOND J. BISHOP, JR., PH.D., certified Rolfer and Rolfing movement instructor, The Center for Inner Work, Sandy Springs, Georgia.

MARGARET MOTHERAL, Certified Massage Therapist, Philadelphia, Pennsylvania.

IRENE O'DAY, R.N., Clinton, Connecticut.

SUSAN POWELL, Atlanta, Georgia.

BARBARA KELLER, Certified Occupational Therapist Assistant (COTA), Short Hills, New Jersey.

BARBARA BORNMANN, M.A., R.D.T., New York, New York.

DIANE JAGOW, R.N., Chelsea, Michigan.

MARY JANE LEE, R.N., Bluemont, Virginia.

SHIRLEY LEVINSON, R.N., C.M.T., Level I and II Reiki practitioner, Coconut Creek, Florida.

LUCY BASLER, ordained minister (Church of the Brethren), hospice chaplain, and therapeutic-touch practitioner, Webster, Wisconsin.

SALLY BLUMENTHAL-MCGANNON, R.N., M.A., L.M.F.T., Aptos, California.

MARIA ARRINGTON, R.N., Bigfort, Montana.

DANIEL J. BENOR, M.D., Holistic Healing Research, Medford, New Jersey.

ROBERT G. BRUCE, III, CLAIRE VAN LEUVEN BRUCE, MICHAEL BOCKENEK, BRITTNYE H. BRUCE, M.S., ASHLEY ELIZABETH BRUCE, DR. LAURA E. MCILWAIN, DR. KIMBERLY L. MCILWAIN, DR. MICHAEL F. MCILWAIN,

A·C·K·N·O·W·L·E·D·G·M·E·N·T·S

SUNJAY DANIEL TREHAN, CHRISTINA YARNOZ, AND HUGH H. CRUSE, M.P.H., for superb research, editing, and marketing skills.

DENISE MARCIL, my agent, for believing in the extraordinary power of touch and for her constant support during the researching and writing phase.

LINDA LOEWENTHAL, SARAH SILBERT, KATHRYN HENDERSON, AND JENNIFER KASIUS, my editors, for intuition, innovation, and personal enthusiasm for this project.

DR. DOLORES KRIEGER, for knowledge and wisdom on the many healing possibilities of human touch.

Contents

CONTENTS

What You Must Know About the Power of Touch

*H*uman touch is a magical and diversified faculty. Its spectrum of sensitivity conveys a wide range of information that encompasses the compacted solidity, flexibility, shape, and texture of physical mass, the probing of its fine edges in the world of nanotechnology, where measure is in fractions of a micron (a human hair's diameter is fifty to one hundred microns), the metaphorical use of the term to connote deep emotion, as in, "You touch me deeply," and in the attempt to describe the further reaches of the nonphysical, as occurs through the hand chakras (Sanskrit: centers of consciousness) of a Therapeutic Touch therapist intent upon healing or helping someone in need. In *Miracle Touch*, Debra Fulghum Bruce brings the therapeutic aspects of this range of touch sensibility to the attention of you, the reader.

Touch, in its many aspects, has intrigued me for most of my adult life. The major avenue of human touch is through the hands. We find that the evolution of the human hand extends to us from out of the further reaches of time. A continuous linkage is unbroken in the recordings of the hand's development. Current neurological thinking is that the hand and the brain evolved together. Crucial and fundamental changes in limb construction occurred as our primordial ancestors learned to travel by swinging from one tree branch to another, and the development of the hand as the body's major manipulative tool and instrument of expression reached through time to include the complex organization of manual skills and the ability to conceive them that active engagement in this modern hi-tech world demands.

A certain recapitulation of form and function can be seen in human embryological development. Neurologically, among the earliest nerve tracts to develop is the spinothalamic, which conveys information to the brain about touch and pain. The spinothalamic nerve tract is protected and made highly efficient by an insulation of fatty myelin tissue that enfolds the tract as a sheath. As the limbs develop and tiny hands find primitive mouth, an active sucking reflex can be seen in early sonographs of the growing fetus. As the fetus comes to term, it experiences repeated cutaneous stimulations during the newborn's descent of the birth canal. Once the baby is born, its further developmental stages derive from a series of touch experiences. Very soon after birth, the baby brings whatever she finds around her to her mouth as she starts to explore her world "out there," her personal environment. At about three months of age, she begins to look at her own hand, an important step in hand-eye coordination. With time, her hand-eye coordination reflexes mature and now she can reach out with mindful purpose and make that world her own.

Touch experiences early in life lay the foundation for later psychological expression or inhibition. The fullness of the touch experience is a uniquely human experience, and its role as probe or antenna for the brain can become sensitively acute as the energies that move the world and its beings now become coherent, patterned, and meaningful. This is apparent, for instance, in the ease with which many people who cannot see learn to read Braille. It is said that as blind persons move their hands over intricately designed indentations and embossments, they learn to visualize in their minds the designs' symbolic content. That is, the hands "read" as though they are stimulus-seeking and information-gathering extensions of the brain.

The hands also describe our emotions and our thinking to ourselves, as when we throw up our hands in exasperation, or count on our fingers to clarify our thinking about quantities. Gestures with the hands convey our innermost thoughts. In Indian traditions certain gestures, called mudras, are considered to be expressions of inner power, often of a spiritual nature. Touch itself can be very expressive. Psychological theory holds that in therapeutic situations, the act of touching a patient means that a therapist is saying to him, "I want to help," and that the patient who allows himself to be touched is replying, "I want to be helped."

In the brain, touch is primarily located in the back of the crown of the head. The largest part of the sensory map we have in the brain is concerned with touch; therefore, touch picks up more data than any of the other senses. Some of the clearest understandings of human touch have come through research that has examined it from the perspective of systems theory. Two outstanding studies currently in progress are under the direction of Gary Schwartz, Ph.D., of the University of Arizona School of Medicine, and Mandayan Srinivasan, Ph.D., of the Massachusetts Institute of Technology. Both of these researchers regard the hands as the major instruments of touch.

Underlying Schwartz' research is a series of hypotheses that focus on patterns of energetic functions of the hands. Called the Hand Energy System Hypotheses, they assume:

1. The hands are a dynamic energy generating system.

2. Energy from the hands may regulate organs and cells in the body interactively.

3. The hands generate patterns of energy. The hand energy pat-

terns include electrical, magnetic, sound, pressure, temperature (infrared), and electrical energies.

4. Hand energy patterns may have interactive effects interpersonally and environmentally, as well as intrapersonally.

5. Levels of consciousness may modulate hand energy patterns in health and illness, and conversely, hand energy patterns may modulate levels of consciousness.

The conceptual framework of touch, therefore, seems to be perceived as multiple, complex, and dynamic energy systems that interact with the fine workings of the body, making known our thoughts and feelings while also manipulating the outer environment. In this, the individual's hands and her levels of consciousness feed back to one another, giving each individual's touch a unique character.

Srinivason, an engineer, considers his study to be in the field of haptics (from the Greek *haptikos*, able to touch). His studies, which probably will be used initially in the field of robotics and computer modeling, use powerful ultrasound devices in the range of fifty megahertz to examine touch sensors in the hand (conventional ultrasound devices that are found in hospitals and other diagnostic centers range from one to ten megahertz). Discussing the hand's neural systems that inform the brain of their sensing, Srinivasan makes the insightful observation that ". . . the hand really ends in the brain," which gives one an appreciation for the multiple relations the hand has to the diverse aspects of human touch.

Natural extensions of these researches pose two important questions for our time: How do electrical impulses translate into perceptions and feelings? What frame of reference would be most effective in an incisive dialogue about human consciousness? So far, the answers have eluded our best minds; however, our culture is beginning to awaken to the importance of such crucial issues. My sense of it is that it will be only as we begin to parse out the answers to such queries that our time will actually enter the "New Age."

A harbinger of this newer age, as Debra Fulghum Bruce will discuss later in this book, is Therapeutic Touch (TT). Therapeutic Touch is a contemporary interpretation of several ancient healing practices that have endured through time. My colleague, Dora Kunz, and I developed TT almost thirty years ago, and we continue to perfect its techniques and sharpen our own understanding of its processes which, in its mature form, are transpersonal in nature. In fact, TT might be called a "no-touch" therapy, for most frequently, the therapist works outside the perimeter of the healee's body, in his nonphysical vital-energy field. However, direct contact can be made with the healee's body, if it is necessary or desired.

Therapeutic Touch has been taught in universities, medical centers, and health agencies in more than ninety foreign countries at the time of this writing. It has been pointed out to me that Therapeutic Touch is a pioneer in its field because it was the first healing modality in the Western world to be taught as a formal part of a fully accredited university curriculum. This occurred at New York University in a masters-level class catalogued as "Frontiers of Nursing" in 1975. The class continues today, and it is a model for other colleges and university courses in Therapeutic Touch in the United States and abroad. At this time, I myself have taught TT to more than 50,000 professional people in the health field and, I'm sure, my students have taught again as many.

Therapeutic Touch has been developed on a foundation of several basic assumptions. The most fundamental of these assumptions is that healing is a natural human potential that can be actualized under appropriate conditions; that is, the ability to help or heal another who is ill, is innate, but slumbering, awaiting each person's individual permission to arise to conscious awareness.

A unique factor of Therapeutic Touch is that the TT therapist begins by centering her consciousness, as do many other modalities. However, in TT the therapist continues in this state of centered consciousness throughout the entirety of the TT process, so that this state of consciousness acts as the constant ground against which the techniques of TT are as figures. Centering entails a distinctive shift in consciousness, during which perception is turned inward in an act of self-exploration to seek out the deeper levels of oneself. As the therapist learns to stay on-center for extended periods of time, she has the opportunity to learn what makes her "tick"; that is, she has the opportunity for self-knowledge and, therefore, insights into one's own self-realization may become embedded in the healing act during the Therapeutic Touch process.

In Therapeutic Touch, touch itself is used as a telereceptor; that is, besides responding to pressure and proprioception, the sense of touch also can pick up information at a distance, as do the other major senses. For example, we taste and smell via chemical molecules floating in the atmosphere, we hear through acoustical pressures, and we see through the intermediary of photons, light waves. All of these major senses act at a distance and, we contend, the sense of touch does similarly.

Therapeutic Touch can finely differentiate between the various vital-energy levels of the individual so that one can recognize changes in the restless, constantly shifting energy patterns that we know most usually only through their functions. The therapist does not always use touch as contact in TT. Nevertheless, as she uses her hands to sense the healee's vital-energy field, usually at a distance of four to six inches from the periphery of the body, the inputs of data become focused, systematized, and explicit in the therapist's mind. We call the appreciation of this information "cues," and what the TT therapist learns about is the therapeutic use of the vital-energy field and the meaning that these cues have for the well-being of the individual healee.

As the TT therapist becomes aware of these cues, in her mind she maps out the characteristics of the healee's vital-energy field, noting areas of energy deficits, significant alterations of vital-energy patterns, critical changes in flow, rhythm, etc. Within the context of Therapeutic Touch, this phase is called the assessment. It is the assessment that informs the next phase, the rebalancing phase of TT. In this phase, the various techniques of TT are used as they are called for by the prior assessment of the healee. From time to time during the rebalancing phase, a reassessment of the healee's vital-energy field is done to get a sense of its current status. The TT therapist knows she has done as much as she can at that time when she can no longer pick up cues. She then terminates the session, and the healee will come back another time, should his condition warrant it.

I have learned that the question that best tells me what it is that TT can do is: What body systems are most sensitive to Therapeutic Touch? Without a doubt, the most sensitive to TT is the autonomic nervous system; therefore, what TT deals very well with is psychosomatic illnesses. This is useful, as psychosomatic illnesses are said to account for at least 70 percent of the health problems in this stress-ladened world.

Only a bit less sensitive are the lymphatic and the circulatory systems, so that Therapeutic Touch works very well and quite quickly with problems of fluid and electrolyte balance. For instance, we have had 4-plus pitting edema significantly reduce in twenty to twenty-five minutes several times, and now we rely upon this action to occur on appropriate occasions. Another reliable effect of TT is a noticeable generalized flush to the skin that indicates the stimulation of the peripheral vascular system. There also appears to be a rapid reaction that occurs to the respiratory system, which seems to be part of a profound relaxation response that occurs within the first four minutes of the session. In this category of sensitivity I would also place the genitourinary system.

On a lower scale of sensitivity, but still of significance, is the musculoskeletal system. In a clinical study several years ago, we were able to x-ray the limbs of persons with bone fractures before, during, and after a series of TT sessions. Particular attention was paid to the extent of callus formation. The average time it took for buildup of strong callus formation under traditional therapies was six weeks; however, with the use of Therapeutic Touch, the average time it took to build up strong, functional callus was two and a half weeks, and that finding has been consistent with subsequent retesting of other samples.

Interestingly, we have had a good response to TT only with certain aspects of other body systems, such as the collagen system, the endocrine system, and the reproductive systems. Clinically the most reliable effects of Therapeutic Touch include:

- A rapid relaxation response that can occur in as little as two to four minutes, with accompanying lowered blood pressure readings, respirations, and pulse rate
- An amelioration or extinction of pain, so that there is a reduced intake of analgesics should any pain persist, and TT also seems to enhance the effects of analgesics already administered
- The healing process itself is facilitated and accelerated, as indicated in the case of bone fractures, as previously mentioned
- TT also facilitates anxiety reduction; for instance, there is relief from nausea, it enhances the rate and rhythm of respirations, and, in all, TT has a profound calming effect

In addition, to a significant extent, Therapeutic Touch promotes:

- A positive change in emotional affect
- The effectiveness of symptoms management in cancer and in AIDS
- A peaceful final transition of those who are terminally ill

Therapeutic Touch uncovers only a small part of the many therapeutic functions of human touch. You have before you a rich source through which you can delve more deeply into this extraordinary spectrum of human function. As I mentioned, throughout my life I have found the study of human touch highly interesting in terms of its versatility, and most challenging in terms of its future potential. I am quite sure that you will find your own search of *Miracle Touch* equally intriguing. Enjoy!

—*Dolores Krieger, Ph.D., RN*
Professor Emerita of Nursing Science
New York University

Miracle
T·O·U·C·H

The Truth About Touch

THE GREATEST SENSE ON OUR BODY IS OUR SENSE OF TOUCH. IT IS PROBA-
BLY THE CHIEF SENSE IN THE PROCESS OF SLEEPING AND WAKING; IT GIVES
US OUR KNOWLEDGE OF DEPTH OR THICKNESS AND FORM; WE FEEL, WE
LOVE AND HATE, ARE TOUCHY AND ARE TOUCHED, THROUGH THE COR-
PUSCLES OF OUR SKIN.

—J. Lionel Taylor

THE STAGES OF HUMAN LIFE

The time was the early 1970s. The Vietnam War had invoked major changes in American society, particularly through the exposure to Eastern Asian culture and the holistic healing practices used there. This exposure, along with the increasing costs and mistrust of our nation's health care, began to fuel the rapid adoption of alternative treatment in the United States.

It was at this time that Dr. Dolores Krieger, a nurse and professor at New York University, along with Dora Kunz, a clairvoyant and healer, became intrigued by the work of healer Oscar Estebany, a Hungarian colonel who was known for curative powers in his healing touch. Krieger did her own experiments on Estebany's patients to see if there really were chemical changes in the body after a therapeutic touch session. The result? Krieger found increased hemoglobin count (the molecule that carries oxygen in the blood) after the session.

Together, Kunz and Krieger, determined that a healing energy field existed, one similar to the Chinese concept of Qi or the East Indian concept of prana, which healers tap into to help people heal themselves. The women proposed that touch was one of the most primitive sensations, and that it had extraordinary efficacy and was worthy of scientific investigation. Since that time, almost thirty years ago, the two healers have been on an extraordinary voyage of unwavering discovery that began a worldwide "touch" movement in the field of nursing.

Today therapeutic touch is not only on the cutting edge of holistic health care, but more than a hundred different types of massage and bodywork—hands-on touch—are skyrocketing in popularity. In fact, more than 85,000 massage therapists provided 25 million Americans with 60 million therapeutic massages in 1998. Massage is now being taught at major universities such as Harvard, Duke, and the University of Miami, and some health-maintenance organizations and insurance companies are recognizing massage therapy as a legitimate health practice.

While the science behind touch therapy is still ambiguous, some theories conclude that healing may occur after a massage or bodywork because of the boost of endorphins and enkephalins (neurochemicals dubbed the "body's natural opiates"), the reduction of the stress hormone cortisol, and the positive change in T cells (the type of lymphocyte responsible for immunity and protection against infection) as immune function improves. Healing touch therapies offer tremendous benefit to people of all ages with all sorts of ailments, including:

+ Alcohol and drug dependency
+ PMS and menopausal symptoms
+ Chronic pain and arthritis
+ Migraine headache
+ Anxiety and depression
+ Asthma, diabetes, and other chronic diseases
+ Repetitive stress injuries
+ Sleep disorders
+ Certain types of cancer
+ HIV and AIDS

HIGH STRESS DEMANDS HIGH TOUCH

Imagine having a deep-muscle-massage "break" instead of a coffee break while you're on the job—and your employer picks up the tab. What about a full-time bodyworker on staff to give "as needed" massages after intense client meetings or tight deadlines? Or perhaps your doctor might prescribe weekly massage therapy instead of pharmaceuticals to help you end insomnia, depression, chronic pain, asthma, smoking cigarettes, or addictions.

As futuristic as this may seem, these are not unrealistic scenarios and are happening in workplaces across the nation. Some experts now contend that our harried lifestyles have caught up with us, and high touch, can help to alleviate the detrimental effects of high-tech stress.

What Is Stress?

Stress describes the many demands—physical, mental, emotional, or chemical—you experience each day. It includes the stressful situation (or stressor) and the symptoms you experience under stress (stress response). Whether stress is negative (distress) or positive (eustress), it is an unavoidable consequence of life. We know from scientific tests that constant stress can wreck your health. In today's pressured society, chronic stress persists for days, weeks, or even months, tearing at your mind, body, and spirit.

What Can It Do?

In reduced productivity, hours lost to absenteeism, and workers'-compensation benefits, stress costs American industry more than $300 billion annually. But more than that, stress can make us ill. That's because cortisol, the body's main stress-related hormone, and the autonomic nervous system are both supercharged during the stress response, commonly called the fight-or-flight response. While these changes can help you fight or flee in an emergency, the physiological changes can tear down your body's ability to ward off illness. As a result of being bathed in stress chemicals, your immune system is no longer able to keep infections or diseases at bay. Consequently, a virus or bacteria can multiply to a point where it infects many cells, eventually giving way to symptoms, disease, and chronic health problems.

Hosts of experiments have shown that if your immune system is strong, exposure to these invaders won't result in health problems. Yet when you are faced with chronic stress, your immune system cannot work at full capacity. When your immune system malfunctions, it yields to the development of autoimmune diseases such as arthritis, allergy, or asthma. If your immune system is depleted, your body is at risk of being overwhelmed by invading bacteria and viruses, which can result in cancer or other life-threatening diseases.

Physical discomfort resulting from psychosocial distress is one of the most common reasons why people seek medical care. A revealing twenty-year study conducted by Kaiser Permanente concluded that over 60 percent of their medical visits were by the "worried well," with no diagnosable medical condition. Not surprisingly, the U.S. Public Health Service estimates that 70 percent of the current health-care budget is spent treating individuals with chronic diseases—many caused by negative lifestyle habits or chronic stress.

What Does It Feel Like?

Your stress response may include the following feelings and behaviors:

- Anger
- Anxiety
- Apathy
- Back pain

+ Chest pain or tightness
+ Colitis
+ Depression
+ Headaches
+ Heart palpitations
+ Hives
+ Impotence
+ Inability to concentrate
+ Inability to relax
+ Insomnia
+ Irregular menstrual period
+ Irritable bowel syndrome (IBS)
+ Loss of sexual desire
+ Loss of sexual function
+ Mood swings
+ Neck pain
+ No or low energy
+ Rapid pulse
+ Short temper
+ Short-term memory loss
+ Weight gain or loss

Not surprisingly, when chronic stress extends over a period of time, you are at risk for the following diseases:

+ Allergies, asthma, and hay fever
+ Backaches
+ Cancer
+ Heart disease
+ High blood pressure
+ Migraine headaches
+ Stroke
+ Tension headaches

- TMJ (temporomandibular joint syndrome)
- Rheumatoid arthritis
- Ulcers

Life's stressors will interrupt you today, tomorrow, and for years to come. While there is no quick fix for coping with stress, you can use healing holistic therapies to help calm your inner turmoil and, subsequently, resolve the deleterious symptoms you may feel. Hands-on touch is one such extraordinary healing therapy. Hands-on touch can not only calm you down after a tumultuous day and heal your inner spirit, it has proven healing benefits that may halt, reverse, or even cure acute or chronic ailments.

WHEN EAST MEETS WEST

Although other alternative-treatment books discuss the myriad of bodywork and touch therapies and outline the necessary how-to steps for health and healing, this book is different. I will tell you the true story of healing touch—how "touch as medicine" evolved from ancient therapies and developed over the centuries into today's New Age trends. I'll report on how people from around the world are using various touch therapies today for physical, emotional, and spiritual healing. One by one, I'll present a multitude of miraculous patient stories, along with some cutting-edge research and therapist interviews. Some of these stories are steeped in scientific substantiation, but most are from people like Ansley Bauer from Dallas, Texas. This thirty-five-year-old librarian was diagnosed with fibromyalgia, an arthritis-like ailment with symptoms of chronic muscle pain, fatigue, and depression.

For three years, Ansley suffered with searing pain in her neck, shoulders, and arms, along with throbbing migraine headaches. She was stiff when she awoke in the mornings and felt continually exhausted, symptoms that she described as flulike. She had not slept well in months, and the more tired she became, the more difficulty she had getting sound sleep. Ansley also had abdominal cramps and diarrhea, followed by bouts of constipation. She had "trigger" points on her back, shoulders, and hips that were tender, and no medicines had given her relief.

When her doctor told her she had fibromyalgia syndrome (FMS), Ansley was thrilled to finally have a diagnosis. But when he added that there was no cure other than to manage the symptoms, her optimism plummeted. After trying various medications with no success, Ansley turned to holistic therapies, including myofascial release, a type of bodywork that involves the application of steady, gentle pressure to the face, neck, and shoulders. The target of this treatment is the fascia—connective tissue that runs throughout the body and has the capacity to impact virtually all joints, muscles, and organs in the body. Myofascial release helps restore motion and eliminate pain in the affected area as imbalances in the body are corrected.

Ansley still has fibromyalgia; there is still no known cure. Yet her symptoms of pain, fatigue, and depression barely exist, and she has returned to an active life. When the FMS symptoms flare, she calls her massage therapist and increases the sessions to twice a week. Healing touch has reversed the path of her chronic and painful ailment, virtually changing her destiny and quality of life.

Throughout my years as a medical writer and author, I've heard testimonies of pain relief, stress relief, resolved depression or anxiety, increased alertness, decreased blood pressure, weight loss, weight gain, and better sleep, all thanks to touch therapy. Some people told about unbelievable cures from drug or alcohol dependency, asthma, hypertension, fibromyalgia, chronic pain, and even cancer with massage, bodywork, or energy-based healing.

But should we accept as fact these personal experiences that are not substantiated in prestigious medical journals? Why not? Even though our medical system is excellent, there are thousands of well-documented accounts of extraordinary healing that most have never read—stories that could change someone else's health and ultimate future. In that regard, *Miracle Touch* moves beyond science to personal testimony. After all, who can question when someone actually feels relief or experiences a cure?

Here's an overview of some of the exciting results; more detailed patient stories appear throughout the book.

- When Cameron hit fifty, he was diagnosed with osteoarthritis in both knees. Rather than giving up his active life and living on anti-inflammatory medications, he found that weekly Swedish massage and moist-heat treatments relieved his joint pain and stiffness enough to increase his activities again. With increased activity, he lost twenty pounds, another boost for reducing arthritis pain and stiffness.

- Fifty-four-year-old Barbara turned to therapeutic touch before and after having gum surgery. The energy-based healing helped to alleviate her anxiety and reduced the need for pain medication after the procedure.

- Ben, twenty-two, found that sports massage helped to increase his athletic prowess on the college baseball field. After a repetitive-stress injury in his shoulder, Ben was back on the playing field within weeks with regular massage therapy.

- After suffering with stress-related headaches for almost a decade, thirty-one-year-old Juanita uses osteopathic manipulation to help ease the pain. Because she has asthma and is allergic to aspirin products, this natural healing treatment gives her excellent relief without causing more problems.

- Bob gets regular acupuncture treatments to help control his alcohol dependency. This forty-year-old attorney finds that the treatments, along with his regular attendance at Alcoholics Anonymous, quell the desire for alcohol and also ease side effects of withdrawal.

- Lynn, thirty-three, uses acupressure and shiatsu for painful menstrual cramps. As a vegetarian, she tries to keep a natural lifestyle, and these ancient Oriental touch therapies keep pain minimal and put Lynn in control of her health.

- When Janelle retired at age sixty-two, she vowed to pamper herself with regular massages. Today, at seventy-two, she uses massage therapy to keep her blood pressure under control. When she interrupts her regular sessions, her blood pressure increases; when she resumes her touch routine, her blood pressure returns to a normal range.

- As an amateur golfer, Stewart relies on chiropractic to stay in alignment. This thirty-two-year-old finds that when he is out of alignment, his golf game is usually off by several points. Stewart's wife, Ellie, twenty-nine, enjoys Swedish massage at a nearby fitness club. She finds the massage helps to keep her muscles supple, especially after lifting weights.

- Sandy, fifty-five, gets Trager and deep-muscle massage when her rheumatoid arthritis flares. As a postmenopausal woman, she believes that the therapies also help to keep her hot flashes and insomnia symptoms controlled.

- Anita gets regular deep-muscle massages to keep her allergies and asthma symptoms at bay. This twenty-three-year-old graduate student has found that a therapeutic massage is particularly helpful during such stressful times as final exams. After a massage, Anita feels relaxed, and her bronchial tubes are not hyperresponsive to allergens or triggers.

* After Rob experienced panic attacks during a live performance, the twenty-seven-year-old singer/songwriter signed up for Feldenkrais training, a bodywork therapy that focuses on improving flexibility, coordination, and range of motion. Using a hands-on form of tactile, kinesthetic communication, the practitioner helped Rob breathe correctly so he would not hyperventilate during times of high anxiety.

* At almost seventy, Sam still goes to the local Y every morning for a one-hour workout. Afterward, he has a massage to reduce pain and increase healing. Sam believes the massage has helped him maintain his excellent muscle tone and allows him to stay active.

Touch therapy can do more than make you feel better; it may even save your life. Ask Stephanie Lowe from Aspen, Colorado, about the lifesaving benefit of massage. Several close friends surprised this forty-year-old mother of three with a spa gift certificate for her birthday. While rubbing sesame oil into Stephanie's skin, the therapist noticed a dark mole on her back and suggested that she ask her doctor to check it. Stephanie hadn't noticed the mole and made an appointment the next day. When the dermatologist saw the mole, he immediately arranged for a biopsy the following week. The result? Stage two melanoma, a skin cancer that, if ignored, could have been deadly. Luckily, the surgeon was able to remove all of the cancer, and Stephanie is fine today, thanks to a very personal "hands-on" massage. She now tells everyone that "a massage is the best birthday present you could give anyone."

A PASSION FOR NATURAL HEALING

As a medical writer, my journalistic passion for truth motivates me to continually seek known and little-known breakthroughs in conventional and alternative treatment to help people ease symptoms or, at best, find a cure for their ailment.

As the author of sixty popular books on health and healing, I've written about some incredible medications and treatments that are virtual lifesavers. I believe touch is equally effective in relieving symptoms of daily stress and reducing problems associated with stress-related ailments. I also believe there are holistic and effective solutions for the millions who suffer daily with stress-related ailments—allergies, asthma, headache, chronic pain, hypertension, gastrointestinal problems, anxiety and depression—and soothing therapies that would help ease the signs and symptoms of serious illness such as cancer or AIDS. As I sought groundbreaking alternative therapies, I found more than I ever imagined—all discussed in this book.

CAN MIRACLE TOUCH HELP YOU?

By now you may be wondering if healing touch and other alternative therapies will help you. There is only one sure way to find out: *Read the book!* Then ask your doctor if these natural holistic therapies may give improvement to your physical and emotional health. The recent profusion of scientific studies on touch therapies has convinced most health-care professionals to support touch as a healing modality—if it causes no harm. (There are some preexisting conditions, such as open wounds, cancer, or vein conditions, that are contraindicated with massage therapy.)

I know that you, too, can feel more alive with the extraordinary healing power of touch. However, the earlier you begin the therapies aimed at your specific problem, the better your results will be. Working with your doctor, make it your goal to become an expert on your body, and then start the healing-touch path to optimal health for the rest of your life.

Let's get started!

CHAPTER ONE

Touch: Help, Hype, or Hoax?

IT IS POSSIBLE THAT HUMAN EMANATIONS EXIST THAT ARE STILL UN-
KNOWN TO US. DO YOU REMEMBER HOW ELECTRICAL CURRENTS AND "UN-
SEEN WAVES" WERE LAUGHED AT? THE KNOWLEDGE ABOUT MAN IS STILL
IN ITS INFANCY.

—*Albert Einstein*

Can a deep-tissue massage really end the chronic pain of migraine headache, arthritis or fibromyalgia syndrome? Will energy-based therapeutic touch help you heal from surgery faster, or ease your anxiety before dental work or other invasive procedures? And can acupuncture, acupressure, or shiatsu be effective treatment for addictions, helping to ease the withdrawal from substance abuse without the need of other heavy medications or in-patient rehabilitation programs?

These are common questions scientists are asking daily as more and more evidence of medical healing touch begins to surface. As one researcher surmised after being personally treated for carpal tunnel syndrome with acupressure, a type of Oriental massage with the fingers, "If seeing is believing, then I've experienced that touching is feeling and healing."

WE EMBRACE ALTERNATIVE THERAPIES

Touching *is* feeling and healing. Yet how many of us long for the physician's calming touch—skin upon skin—whether with a firm handshake, a compassionate pat on the back, or an assuring hand on the shoulder? Tired of assembly-line medical care where doctors spend an average of ten minutes per patient at each visit, many seek natural and effective ways to prevent, manage, or even cure diseases, using methods that are often not scientifically based. This alternative medical care is tagged "drug-free doctoring," since it views the mind and body as a totally integrated system. This means they influence each other and depend on your self-care to stay well.

The skyrocketing use of complementary medicine indicates a growing dissatisfaction with conventional or allopathic health care. Allopaths, or conventional medical doctors, define disease based on measurable symptoms and try to eliminate those signs; alternative therapists treat the whole person—body, mind, and spirit—with a focus on staying balanced and well.

Although many alternative healers, including touch-therapy practitioners, do not have medical degrees or official recognition from the American Medical Association (AMA), people are turning to these alternative therapies in droves. Why? Because they are appealing, and they offer hope, which is often the missing ingredient in the healing equation. Especially with the soaring costs of health care, alternative touch treatments, which range from massage to traditional Chinese medicine to energy-based medicine, are relatively affordable, easily accessible, and allow you to participate actively in key decisions about your health.

PROOF IS TRUTH

While some people embrace alternative therapies, others demand proof that something works. "Show me the science," Dr. Randall Briggs, a twenty-five-year orthopedist from the Midwest, said when asked if deep-muscle massage might heal a patient's arthritic joints. Yet Briggs also admitted that at least once a week, a patient claims healing after massage therapy.

Lynn's Incredible Cure
Massage Stopped the Deep Muscle Pain of Fibromyalgia

Extensive studies have shown that massage, in particular, reduces anxiety and lowers the body's production of stress hormones. That healing response gives a significant benefit to someone like thirty-nine-year-old Lynne Teague, a real estate broker from South Florida who was diagnosed with a chronic arthritis-related syndrome that causes deep muscle pain. "I went to four different doctors over a period of two years to find out what was causing the deep muscle pain and chronic fatigue," Lynne said.

"Three of the doctors told me the pain was in my head. But I knew differently. The last doctor did a series of tests and reviewed my symptoms and medical history. Then he went one step further to seek an accurate diagnosis. He carefully touched different trigger points [specific spots on the body that are painful to touch] and confirmed that I had fibromyalgia. He said there was no treatment other than to minimize the symptoms.

"I asked him about bodywork. He shrugged his shoulders, laughed, then mumbled something about needing to check on his car at the mechanic's shop. He then told me there was not much science to back up bodywork for fibromyalgia muscle pain. Sick and tired of feeling sick and tired, I decided to try touch therapy anyway.

"When I went to the appointment at a nearby massage-therapy center, I was impressed at how professional everyone was. The receptionist asked me to fill out a medical history form, then one of the therapists took me in a room to give me some background. I didn't realize the therapists were licensed after taking a two-year program and undergoing twenty-two hundred hours of practical training.

"Another massage therapist took me into a small room that was painted a very soothing blue. I remember there was classical music playing in the background, and aromatherapy candles were burning near the windowsill. The therapist showed me to a dressing area where I exchanged my street clothes for a long white sheet, which I discreetly tucked around my body.

"I sat on the long table, and the therapist began to rub sweet-smelling sesame oil on my skin, then she softly kneaded my tightened muscles. Using a gentle, rocking motion, the therapist began to release tension out of my upper body and then had me lie down facing the table. Her hands worked up and down my painful trigger points. Sometimes I felt like her fingers were pointing right into my skin, but she said that's where my muscles were so tense. She focused mostly on my upper body—my neck, shoulders, and upper back—where my pain was the worst.

"After the massage, I was almost afraid to move. I was relaxed, and the pain was almost nonexistent. Finally, as I was getting dressed, I realized that the range of motion in my arms was greater and the tension in my upper body was greatly reduced. I continued receiving thirty-minute massages twice a week for six months and had greatly reduced pain and stiffness, less fatigue, and less difficulty sleeping. While my medical doctor gave me the accurate diagnosis, it was human touch that gave me a normal life again."

TOUCH CAN CURE SYMPTOMS AND SOME DISEASES

Could healing touch be the new cure you've been longing for to end nagging health concerns? While some feel that a cure means complete healing of the symptoms and disease, *Stedman's Medical Dictionary*, disagrees: A cure is "a restoration to health; a special method or course of treatment." Certainly there are a host of diseases that baffle medical researchers; however, the touch therapies described in this book have worked for millions around the world to reduce or even end symptoms, without side effects.

Through comprehensive scientific research, we know that tactile stimulation is necessary for the arousal and development of various physiological systems and is fundamentally required for healthy relationships—but what about healing touch as a viable form of medical treatment? Is it hype, hoax, or actual healing? Granted, it feels comforting to be touched. Who doesn't benefit from a friend's warm hug, a pat on the back for a job well done, or a newborn baby nestled on your neck? But can human touch actually bring about physiological changes in the body that we associate with healing? Yes! We also know the opposite is true—a touchless society can lead to failure to thrive and even death in newborn babies.

"No Touch" Leads to Failure to Thrive

The perils of a touchless society became apparent in the early 1900s, when Dr. Luther Emmett Holt, known as one of America's first and finest pediatricians, decided that parents were spoiling their children by cuddling and holding them too much. Good parents took notice and immediately followed his order, beginning a trend of hands-off parenting. Within just a few years, doctors across the nation started to notice a dramatic increase in infant deaths—particularly in seemingly healthy babies. It soon became apparent that these infants failed to thrive simply because they were not getting enough human contact. There are hosts of studies concluding that infants who suffered from touch deprivation in orphanges achieved only half of the height normal for their age.

In touch studies done on animals, monkey infants who were denied contact—a "secure base"—ceased to explore their environments. Research in animal behavior also reveals that when animals are deprived of touch, they become aggressive and violent.

Touch Boosts Preemie Growth

We have come a long way in understanding the importance of touch with human development. In support of touch boosting immune system function, a host of researchers have reported decreased cortisol, and increased numbers and activity of natural killer-cell activity following massage therapy. Natural killer cells are immune-system cells that are important in killing virus-infected cells and cancer cells. For children with chronic diseases, touch can alleviate symptoms and let them live a more normal life. In fact, researchers say fifteen minutes of massage a day can help a diabetic child's glucose levels remain in the normal range and improve an asthmatic child's pulmonary functions.

Touch Influences Emotional Development

Further studies show a strong link between touch and emotional development. Infants of the Netsilik Inuit tribe of the Canadian Arctic are very calm and cry very little. This is thought to be because they are almost constantly carried on their mothers' backs and can communicate with them through touch. In one study done at the Child Development Program at Montreal Children's

---

Ongoing Trials at the Renowned Touch Research Institute

Promising studies by Dr. Tiffany Fields, a Miami child psychologist, and her colleagues at the University of Miami's Touch Research Institute confirm that massage stimulates the vagus nerves, which then trigger processes that aid digestion, among other things. According to Fields, as a result of their speedy weight gain, massaged preemies are discharged to their parents an average of six days earlier, shaving $10,000 off their hospital tab. With four hundred thousand premature babies born in the U.S. every year, the potential cost savings are obvious. And eight months after birth, massaged preemies have superior motor skills and mental development. Full-term infants and older babies also benefit from touch and massage.

Parenting Expert Believes Touch Stimulates Newborn's Breathing

Dr. William Sears, renowned pediatrician, author, and staunch advocate of "attachment parenting," believes parents who spend time touching their babies—skin to skin—help them to thrive and develop physically, emotionally, and intellectually. "Attachment parenting involves what I call the five Baby B's—birth bonding, breast-feeding, baby wearing, bedding close to baby, and belief in baby's cries. Skin-to-skin contact is vital for making this connection with baby and helps parents to know their infants and become experts in their baby's needs. Besides being enjoyable, stroking the skin is medically beneficial to the newborn. The skin, the largest organ in the human body, is very rich with nerve endings. At the time when baby is making the transition to air breathing, and the initial breathing patterns are very irregular, stroking stimulates the newborn to breathe more rhythmically, giving a parent's touch real therapeutic value."

Hospital, researchers asked volunteer mothers to carry their babies for at least three hours a day. They then compared the babies' crying patterns with those of a group who weren't carried. The babies who were held more cried less.

A TOUCH/PHOBIC SOCIETY

Although touch allows us to unwind and heal our inner spirit, confusion surrounds its curative powers. Some people shy away from this centuries-old healing modality, especially Americans, who, unlike the rest of the world, have been reared to avoid touch, fearing that it's "sleazy" and will encroach on another's private space.

"Disrobe before a stranger just to get a massage? I don't think so." Forty-nine-year-old Miranda Peters from Nashville, Tennessee, says what many still believe—touch from a stranger is too intimate and often quite intimidating. Phyllis Davis, a licensed professional counselor, says that most Americans have an eighteen-inch boundary separating them from another person. In a two-person conversation, if one participant moves closer to the other, he or she immediately responds by backing away. In a revealing study, researchers observed couples in cafés and restaurants across the globe and tallied the following dismal (if you are an American) results:

- Puerto Ricans touch an average of 180 times per hour.
- The French touch 110 times per hour.
- Americans touch 2 times an hour.

In another key study reported in the journal *Adolescence* (Winter 1999), Dr. Tiffany Fields and the Touch Research Institute, along with researchers from Nova Southeastern University in Fort Lauderdale, Florida, observed forty adolescents at McDonald's restaurants in Paris, France, and Miami, Florida, to assess the amount of touching and aggression during their peer interactions. The scientists noted that the American teenagers spent less time leaning against, stroking, and hugging their peers than did the French adolescents. Researchers observed that the American teens showed more self-touching and more aggressive verbal and physical behavior.

The Most Significant Diagnostic Tool

"Perhaps the most significant diagnostic instrument in the world is the human hand attached to the human mind. In medicine, a doctor's touch saves lives. The doctor can make a life-saving diagnosis after feeling lymph nodes, abdominal masses, breast lumps, rhythm of irregular pulses, and the texture of a skin lesion.

While the use of gloves in medicine is good from a hygienic standpoint, it is bad from a diagnostic and rapport standpoint. That thin millimeter layer of latex makes a large difference."

Joel C. Silverfield, M.D.,
rheumatologist with
Tampa Medical Group, P.A.

HIPPOCRATES AFFIRMED TOUCH AS A HEALING MODALITY

If people claim healing from various hands-on therapies, then why is touch so avoided in our high-tech society that prides itself in seeking the best of all healing traditions? After all, it was Hippocrates (around 460 B.C.) who described the healing power of the "force that flows from many people's hands." The father of medicine also wrote: "The physician must be experienced in many things, but most assuredly in rubbing" (the Greek and Roman term for massage).

For centuries, physicians' hands were their most important diagnostic and therapeutic tools. Today, however, most conventional medical practitioners refrain from physical contact with the patient and lean toward diagnostic equipment because of legal and time variables. As one medical doctor said, "There is just no scientific substantiation that rubbing a back will completely halt the pain caused by a pulled muscle, joint pain, or herniated disk. Besides, I would face malpractice if I touched someone and she felt it was inappropriate."

But isn't the skin a vital part of the body—a part that must be felt to check on its health? Some experts claim that of all the senses to lose, the sense of touch is the most precious. After all, the skin is your body's largest sense organ, and all forms of touch are perceived through the skin. While other senses—hearing, smell, sight, and taste—diminish with age, the need for touch actually increases.

As the body's outer covering, your skin protects you against heat, light, injury, and infection and is sensitive to many different kinds of stimuli, such as pain, pressure, temperature, and joint and muscle position sense (called proprioception). The skin regulates your body temperature and stores water, fat, and vitamin D.

Your sense of touch originates in the bottom layer of the skin, or the dermis. The dermis is filled with many tiny nerve endings that give you information about the things with which your body comes in contact. Your body has about twenty different nerve endings in the skin, which tell you if something is hot, cold, or going to hurt you. The nerve endings convey this information to the brain and spinal cord, also known as the central nervous system (CNS), to areas where we perceive the stimuli. To accomplish this, the nerve endings of the sensory receptors convert mechanical, thermal, or chemical energy into electrical signals.

WHAT HAPPENS WHEN WE ARE TOUCHED?

In his book *Subtle Energy: Awakening to the Unseen Forces in Our Lives* (Warner Books, 1998), William Collinge, Ph.D., tells of some fascinating breakthroughs discovered at the Institute of HeartMath. Collinge describes one particular study in which researchers Rollin McCraty and his colleagues wanted to find out whether the heart energy fields are measurable at the surface of the body when we are in close proximity or actually touching. The study involved wiring pairs of subjects to electrodes and placing them five feet apart. The researchers realized that the electrodes did not identify one person's heart energy waves (electrocardiogram output) on the surface of the other person's body at that distance. Yet, when the subjects touched hands, each person's heart energy waves were measurable on the surface of the other's body and even in the other's brain waves.

In another similar experiment, Collinge gives details of how the researchers sought to determine whether heart energy was transferred when the subjects were sitting even closer—yet still not touching. With the subjects' bodies wired with electrodes, electrocardiogram output was detectable on the surface of each other's bodies—even though the subjects were spaced three feet apart. The researchers concluded that the heart energy field—the most powerful electromagnetic field of the human body—is both conducted by physical contact and radiated across space between people.

When we touch another person, there appears to be a real transfer of energy. Examples of well-known energies are light, heat, the temperature of our body or of a room, sound, and kinetic energy, which keeps our hearts beating. We use kinetic energy to stand, sit down, shout, whisper, and breathe. Subtle energies are involved in any energy-based healing. These are the very emotions that make up our thoughts and feelings, including anxiety, fear, determination, frustration, anger, hope, exultation, emotional pain, worry, and excitement.

ENERGY-BASED HEALING

Unlike massage, which is hands-on healing, therapeutic touch is based on the assumption that a human energy field extends beyond the skin. The idea behind TT is that this energy field is abundant and flows in balanced patterns in health but is depleted or unbalanced in illness or injury. Practitioners work to restore health by sensing and adjusting such fields. Proponents say therapeutic touch can heal wounds, relieve tension headaches, reduce stress and pain, and facilitate the body's natural restorative processes.

Easing the Final Journey
Therapeutic Touch Gave a Dying Woman Peace

Diane Connors, a sixty-one-year-old registered nurse and hospice caseworker from Phoenix, has used therapeutic touch frequently and finds it valuable in easing anxiety, nausea, pain, and respiratory distress. This veteran health-care professional tells of a time when she was scheduled to visit a dying patient. "This woman was young, beautiful, and brilliant, and she was being admitted to hospice with advanced metastatic breast cancer.

"When I heard her voice, it was so vibrant with its rich French accent, but the words were desperate as she reached out in fear and angst. She knew she was dying, but her heart was broken for the life she was leaving—a compassionate husband and preschool-age daughter. She didn't want to go—not just yet.

"As I tended to her physical needs, I spoke with her about her life, her family, and the dreams she had. She talked openly, cried softly, and even laughed as we spoke. She readily accepted the offer of therapeutic touch, and after doing this for thirty minutes, she lay in her bed peacefully. She no longer felt physical pain, her face was glowing, and she expressed love and gratitude to her husband for their life together.

"This was the first and last time I saw this woman. When I returned to hospice three days later, I was told that she had died in her sleep. Then hospice received this in a letter from her husband: 'The nurse arrived, spoke to her with caring and understanding, artfully attended her needs, and then calmed her very noticeably by using a "no-touch therapy," which we had never before witnessed. My wife remained at peace and was calm until she died. For that I am grateful.' "

Healing Touch Realigns Energy Flow

Healing Touch (HT), sponsored by the American Holistic Nurses Association, is another energy medicine. This complementary mode functions from an energy perspective rather than a physical one. The Healing-Touch practitioner realigns the energy flow, reactivating the mind/body/spirit connection to eliminate blockages to self-healing. Healing Touch International certifies registered nurses, physicians, body therapists, counselors, psychotherapists, and other health professionals and individuals desiring an in-depth understanding and practice of healing work using energy-based concepts.

Reiki Utilizes Energy to Trigger Healing

Like Healing Touch, Reiki utilizes the energy force to trigger health and healing. Reiki, or universal life energy, is thought to have been used by Tibetan monks thousands of years ago, yet the practice of Reiki was lost through the generations. Dr. Mikao Usui rediscovered this age-old healing modality in the mid-nineteenth century and began to teach it throughout Japan.

Randy's Long-Awaited Healing
"After Reiki I Regained My Strength and Will to Live Again"

Randy Petersen, a thirty-four-year-old Level II Reiki practitioner from Oakland, California, has been studying this alternative form of medicine since he was in an automobile accident more than a decade ago.

"After my car accident, I was in bad shape. I had broken my leg in two places and had superficial wounds all over my face and arms. But not only was I in pain and immobile, I became very depressed. I didn't think I'd ever get beyond the limitations I had.

"One of my colleagues, Elizabeth, came to see me after I got home. She was greatly distressed that I was so despondent and without my usual enthusiasm and vigor for life. Elizabeth asked if she could try using Reiki on me. I had heard of Reiki from some friends but had never received this personally.

"After saying a prayer, Elizabeth very gently touched the different parts of the body, beginning at the top of my head with my eyes and then moving in an intricate pattern all the way down to the feet. She then did some movements without hands-on touch, sort of like a full-body massage, yet there was no rubbing.

"Throughout the session, I felt a static or electric sensation, much like pins and needles when a part of the body is said to have fallen asleep. Elizabeth worked on my body for more than thirty minutes, then covered me with a light blanket. I fell asleep instantly and was so relaxed. It was after that session that I regained some strength and my will to get well again."

Reiki practitioners claim that when the negativity is released from the body, it may take various forms, including chills, warmth, twitches, drowsiness, laughter, crying, or dreams.

The Emotional Side of Touch

Beyond the physical healing that is attributed to hands-on and energy-based touch therapies, there is a deeper emotional side that tugs at the very core of our existence: Positive touch makes us feel

---

A Physician Realizes That Touch Is Medicine

"In my first few days as an intern at Yale–New Haven Hospital, and as a young and naive physician, I found myself explaining to a newly admitted patient with unexplained pain that she was in one of the nation's truly great hospitals. With Yale–New Haven's superb laboratories, consultants, and brainpower at hand, we would surely find out what was wrong and that she would certainly get well.

"At first there was some understanding, even acceptance, of what I was saying. Yet there was little comfort for the patient. I'm not a person prone to causal physical contact, but I instinctively bent over, gently touched her arm, and told her that I would take care of her. For some reason, I was never

comfortable enough, or perhaps my ego wasn't strong enough, to do this before.

"Immediately, a gentle peace developed across this patient's face. At that time, I viewed myself as the lowest person in that medical mecca, but when I saw the relief this patient was feeling, I knew I was practicing medicine.

"To this day, I don't remember her name or even her final diagnosis. But I do recall that she quickly improved and was discharged after several days."

—*Samuel S. Thatcher, M.D., Ph.D., reproductive endocrinologist and author of* POLYCYSTIC OVARY SYNDROME: THE HIDDEN EPIDEMIC *(Perspectives Press, 2000).*

good and calms our inner spirit. A growing body of evidence points to the following conclusions: When one person touches another in a noncontroversial manner, it results in a positive reaction. When you are touched by a loved one, your thoughts can range from erotic to endearing to comforting. While modern science cannot measure what you feel, almost everyone has felt the hope of human touch.

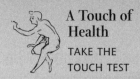
Touch Makes You Feel Loved

The ability that physical feelings have to transmit emotional feelings is incredible. Judith Goldberg, a forty-two-year-old licensed marriage and family counselor from Manhattan, shared: "I was talking with a mother and her fifteen-year-old daughter recently. I asked the mother if her daughter loved her, and she replied, 'Oh, certainly.' Then I asked the teenager if she felt that her mother loved her, to which she replied, 'No, she doesn't.' The mother was

It's Not That Funny!

While a surprise tickle from a friend may cause barrels of laughter, scientists have found you cannot tickle yourself. The cerebellum, at the back of the brain, ignores expected sensations and tells your brain, "Ah, don't get excited. It's just you!"

Your brain knows to predict what you will feel when you or your body does something. This mechanism lets you ignore certain touch sensations

like the weight or pressure on the soles of your feet while you walk. Your brain saves the alert for times when you step on a piece of glass or a sharp rock.

Research published in the journal *Nature Neuroscience* (November 1998) concluded that during self-tickling, the cerebellum tells an area called the somatosensory cortex what to expect, and this dampens the tickling sensation.

shocked by her statement and said, 'I tell you I love you every day.'
The teen responded, 'But you never hug me . . .' "

Virginia Satir, a family clinician, researcher, and seminal theorist who deepened our understanding of psychology and relationships has said that unless we get about a dozen hugs a day, we risk
having our spirit die. Satir believed people needed four hugs a day
for survival, eight for maintenance, and twelve for growth.

Touch Elicits Positive Feelings

A study at a midwestern university library adds credence to the
affect of touch on impression formation. Half of the students who
came into the campus library were briefly touched on the forearm
or hand by the librarian or assistants as they checked out books.
The other students were not touched at all. After the students left
the library, they were all asked to rate their overall impression of
the library services. All of the students who were touched had
positive feelings about the library and staff. The students who
were not touched had negative or apathetic statements.

Touch Boosts Healing

"Kangaroo care" is yet another proven touch method used to stabilize premature infants and boost healing. This term describes
skin-to-skin contact with parents and other caregivers. The infant, wearing only a diaper and covered by a blanket, is placed
against the parent's bare chest. Proponents of kangaroo care claim
the method has amazing effects: a steadier heart rate, better
breathing, greater contentment, and restful sleep.

There is a story of infant twins who were separated at birth:
Each was placed in her respective incubator because one was not
expected to live. Believing that the babies belonged together, a
nurse at the hospital fought against hospital rules and placed both
infants in one incubator. When they were placed together, the
healthier of the two threw an arm over her sister in an endearing

embrace. The smaller baby's heart rate stabilized and her temperature rose to normal. The twins survived their rocky beginning and in time went home with their parents. Later, a photo of this famous embrace, called "Rescuing Hug," appeared both in *Life* and *Reader's Digest*.

THE JURY IS IN

While there are endless cases of self-reported healing, scientists are not usually satisfied unless the results can be measured with laboratory equipment. It's almost impossible to measure how you feel when someone gives you a hug. What about the release of stress you feel after a full-body massage? Or what causes that warm "pins and needles" sensation that many receive after a therapeutic-touch session? In most cases, the only one who can measure healing results is the patient herself.

Touch Reduces Stress Hormones

Some researchers have identified, at least in part, a physiological basis for the behavioral effects of touch-deprived animal infants. Stress hormones, in particular, appear to play a key role. In studies on rhesus monkeys reared by peers rather than their mothers, researchers found abnormal stress hormone responses to a variety of stressors. Many experts contend the same outcome holds true for humans, too.

Touch Blocks Opportunistic Disease

It's becoming more and more apparent to even the most skeptical scientist that touch does have an effect on the parasympathetic nervous system, the calming system that conserves the body's energy, and that it also induces the production of endorphins, the body's natural pain-killing hormones that help to keep the adrenal glands from being overly stressed. To show this dramatic connec-

Geriatric Specialist Finds That Touch Gives Comfort

"Of all the treatments I use, human touch is guaranteed to give comfort. So many of my colleagues believe that if they didn't learn it in medical school or see proof in a published study, then it's not true. I disagree. I believe that if a treatment works and causes no harm—whether conventional or alternative—then it should be considered.

"Recently, during my regular visit to a nearby retirement village, I stopped to check on my patient Anna. This eighty-nine-year-old woman was in chronic pain from arthritis and usually stayed to herself because of the discomfort.

"This one day, as I rubbed my hand over the elderly woman's arthritic wrist, I couldn't help but notice a faint smile appear on her face. Knowing her history, I don't think the manipulation of her tiny bones did anything magical

to alleviate the ravages of her pain. But being in a nursing home, Anna was devoid of human touch, except for an occasional nurse feeling her pulse upon awakening each day or another patient pushing her out of his way in the cafeteria. As I gently rubbed her tiny wrist, I could sense her feeling of relief that someone cared.

"When I returned to the nursing home the next week, Anna was sitting on the couch in the TV lounge with two friends—all three women reached out to me with their frail, arthritic wrists, longing for the healing power of human touch."

—Dr. Harris McIlwain, a Florida-based rheumatologist, geriatric specialist, and author of fifteen books, including THE FIBROMYALGIA HANDBOOK *(Holt, 1999) and* THE OSTEOPOROSIS CURE *(Avon, 1998)*

tion, researchers have conducted a number of immune studies with monkeys to test the relationship between physical contact and the body's ability to respond to an immunological challenge (in this case, a tetanus shot). They found a direct relationship between the amount of contact and the amount of grooming an infant received in the first six or seven months of life and its ability to produce antibodies, proteins called immunoglobulins that are part of the body's natural defense mechanism and neutralize foreign proteins in the body, in response to an antibody challenge at a little over a year of age. Their conclusion? Human touch serves as a preventive measure for blocking opportunistic disease.

Touch Is Valuable in Miraculous Healing

Scientists at the Touch Research Institute believe touch not only aids in preventing disease but offers many possibilities in human healing:

- Surgical wounds and sutures heal faster
- Burns clear up sooner
- Circulation and breathing improve postsurgically
- Enhances the growth rate of premature infants
- Lowers the stress hormones cortisol and norepinephrine, which are thought to diminish the effects of the immune system
- Increases the production of serotonin (a brain chemical that is related to pain and mood) and of endorphins, the body's natural painkillers
- Improves blood circulation

Touch Is the Missing Link in Medicine Today

Imagine being in a large noisy room, like a train station or airport, and people dressed in stark, white uniforms are bustling in various directions focused on their specific tasks. Now envision that you are lying on a hard hospital bed while some stranger sticks your arm intermittently to get blood or to find an IV site.

As a doctor, I always think how utterly inhumane patients must feel when they come to the hospital for emergency care. Yet I've found that if I immediately hold their hands or touch their arms while examining them, they quickly look up into my eyes with a sense of ultimate trust. Then the next time I walk into their hospital room, these patients have made a human connection and immediately extend their hands to touch mine. Even without speaking, I convey through touch that I'll try my hardest to get them well. Perhaps touch is the missing link in medicine today that can greatly improve a patient's outcome.

—Kimberly McIlwain, M.D.

- Lowers blood pressure and heart rate
- Boosts the body's immune system, which promotes fast healing
- Improves growth and development in premature babies
- Improves breathing function in children and adults with asthma as it increases relaxation

COMFORT, HOPE, AND HEALING

By now you may be wondering if touch therapies will ease your symptoms or even help you destress, sleep sounder, or enjoy life more fully. There is only one way to find out: Read about the many types of touch therapies in this book, then see if they may help your situation. Especially in today's fast-paced, rapidly changing, high-pressure world, touch therapies may give you the much needed comfort, hope, and healing we all long for.

CHAPTER TWO

Steeped in Ancient Traditions

TOUCH IS THE MOTHER OF ALL SENSES.

—*Ashley Montague*

So much myth and misinformation surround touch therapies that most people are unaware of the age-old roots. Even though there are ancient writings from Egypt, Persia, Greece, Rome, and Asian countries that all mention the positive effects from the use of massage, many historians speculate that massage or touch therapies began as a medical treatment in China.

THE FORCES OF YIN AND YANG

Chinese medicine is as old as Chinese civilization itself and gets its theoretical basis from the Taoist principles of yin and yang, the five movements or seasons of life, which describe a continual cycle of energy—rising, falling, and rising again, and "Qi" (pronounced "chi"), the body's vital energy. The significance of yin and yang has infiltrated every part of Chinese existence since the earliest of recorded time, influencing astrology, medicine, art, and even government. Thought to be complementary forces or principles, yin and yang make up all aspects of life; their literal translation is "bright side/dark side." Yin is like earth, female, dark, passive, and absorbing; it is represented by the tiger, the color orange, and a

Since the third century B.C. in China, yin and yang have permeated thought. Even today they are associated with having lucky or unlucky days or considering the zodiac before making a decision.

broken line. Yang is thought to be like heaven, male, light, and active. Yang is present in odd numbers and is represented by the dragon, the color azure, and an unbroken line.

When the body is in balance between yin and yang, health is predominant; when the yin and yang are imbalanced, disease occurs. Chinese medicine practitioners view yin and yang as a way of seeing life: All things work together to be part of a whole; nothing is seen in isolation or as absolute. This philosophy of healing is contrary to Western medicine, where a specific disease may be treated separately without considering the total health of the person—mind, body, and spirit.

Balancing the Five Elements

The concept of yin and yang is associated in Chinese with the idea of the five agents (or elements), including metal, wood, water, fire, and earth. The goal of the Chinese practitioner is to harmonize yin and yang and restore balance through these elements. Taoists have studied the elements' relationships and devised a system of references enabling them to understand the world, including all aspects of life.

Qi Is the Life Force

Along with yin and yang, Qi forms the basis for Chinese healing, or external Qi healing, since it encompasses the meaning of all vital activities and substances in the human body. Qi is the life force of all living things and represents all energy within the universe. It is the source of movements, ranging from blood flow to voluntary muscle action; it protects your body from external interruptions, and it generates warmth for the body.

HOW DOCTORS TREAT DISEASE

The concept behind traditional Chinese medicine is very progressive. Not only is it highly personal, but it was one of the first traditions to grasp the potential within the broader field of preventive medicine. In earlier days in China, a doctor was paid to keep a person healthy. As soon as a person became ill, he got his treatment for free. Conventional Western medicine presupposes that disease results from an external force, such as a virus or bacteria, or a degeneration of the body's functional ability. Symptoms are treated using pharmaceuticals or invasive surgery. Conversely, Chinese doctors treat the entire body, not a specific complaint or symptom. Helping "good" Qi to chase away "bad" Qi, doctors work to boost patient healing and minimize any side effects. Chinese doctors believe that Western medicine is too self-limiting because of its need to back up procedures and treatments with strong science.

Pathways Through the Body

Qi travels along twelve imaginary meridians (also called pathways or channels) to keep the body nourished. These meridians start at your fingertips, connect to the brain, and then to the organ associated with the specific meridian. The twelve regular meridians correspond to specific human organs: kidneys, liver, spleen, heart, lungs, pericardium, bladder, gallbladder, stomach, small and large intestines, and the triple burner (body-temperature regulator).

Yin meridians flow up; yang meridians flow down. Pathways corresponding to the yang organ are often used to treat disorders of its related yin organ. For example, the lung meridian is connected to the lungs via the nervous system. Theoretically, a lung problem will arise if there is an obstruction in the lung meridian that slows down the flow of energy. When Qi is blocked or thrown off balance, illness or symptoms result. If you have pain, or "Bi," from a torn or injured muscle, traditional Chinese medicine says that the channel running through the damaged muscle has been physically disrupted, resulting in local pain or a disease of Bi. To treat this, the flow of energy through the channel must be restored using acupuncture, acupressure, or other ancient therapies.

THE HEALING POWER OF ACUPRESSURE

What Is It?

Surely you've spontaneously grabbed your temples when your head is pounding, or rubbed your abdomen when you ate too much. This touching of certain points on the body is a natural reaction, and it's the foundation of acupressure. This popular form of Chinese healing uses touch to unblock Qi and allow the meridians or pathways to flow smoothly.

Where Did It Come From?

Most people are familiar with acupuncture, the insertion of needles in the body for treatment of disease. Acupressure was actually discovered before acupuncture and uses the same bodily points but no needles. It was virtually neglected after the Chinese developed acupuncture because they thought the use of needles was a more technological method for stimulating points.

How Does It Work?

Using gentle pressure, this hands-on therapy is applied with the thumb or index finger at specific trigger points on the body. On the physical level, acupressure affects muscular tension, blood circulation, and other physiological parameters. Traditional Oriental healing believes that the stimulation of these trigger points releases energy or unblocks Qi, resulting in health and healing. Scientific researchers find that both acupressure and acupuncture cause the body to release endorphins and monoamines, chemicals that block pain signals in the spinal cord and the brain. The endorphin system consists of chemicals that regulate the activity of a group of nerve cells in the brain that relax muscles, dull pain, and reduce panic and anxiety. The system can also lower blood pressure and reduce the heart's workload. These ancient touch therapies may also trigger the release of more hormones, including serotonin, a brain chemical that makes you feel calm and serene, as well as the anti-inflammatory chemical known as cortisol. The benefits also include increased circulation and decreased tension.

These points (more than fifteen hundred of them) are all along the meridians. When a practitioner touches one of these points, he or she refers healing to another part of the body. For example, a point on your second toe is used to treat headaches and toothaches; a point near your elbow helps to boost immune function.

During treatment, each point is held with a steady pressure for one to three minutes, using the tips or balls of the fingers or thumb. If the acupressure point is sensitive or tender, this indicates that the meridian (energy pathway or channel) is blocked. During the treatment, this tenderness should dissipate as the channel becomes unblocked and energy flows freely again.

What's It Good For?

Today acupressure exists mainly in Asian countries like India, China, Japan, and Korea and is used to relieve everyday aches, pains, and stress, as well as specific conditions like sinus pressure, leg cramps, headaches, temporomandibular joint disorder (TMJ), which causes pain in the jaw and ear, and carpal tunnel syndrome.

Acupressure can also be combined with massage to release tension, increase circulation, reduce pain, and develop optimal health.

Using regular acupressure helps to trigger the relaxation response, a physiological state characterized by a feeling of warmth and quiet mental alertness. Practitioners believe that it may help to counteract the debilitating effects of stress so your brain waves shift from an alert beta rhythm to a relaxed alpha rhythm. Acupressure helps to summon this state because it is active touching.

Many touch therapists experience reduced blood pressure after they give a massage, no matter how strenuous the strokes were. When you are actively involved in "doing," your mind cannot focus on the worries of the moment. It's quite difficult to worry about your bills or your career when you are concentrating on specific acupressure points!

Where's the Science?

In a study reported by the *American Journal of Hypertension* (May 2000), researchers at Maimonides Medical Center in Brooklyn, New York, found that acupressure and acupuncture helped to lower blood pressure. While the findings are preliminary, those participants with essential hypertension who underwent four weeks of acupressure and acupuncture therapy had lower blood pressure and greater stress release than patients who were not treated. Researchers look to further studies to address the mechanism by which the therapies lower blood pressure.

A Touch of Health

USE ACUPRESSURE TO END LEG CRAMPS

Try acupressure to end annoying leg cramps. Using two fingers, press the point on the back of your leg in the center of the base of the calf muscle. This point is midway between the crease behind the knee and the heel. Hold for forty-five seconds for optimum relief.

Britt's Remarkable Pain Cure
Acupressure Stopped Chronic Pain and Gave Britt Her Life Back

After twenty-nine-year-old Britt Taylor, a high school biology teacher from San Diego, California, was injured in a serious car accident, she lived with constant pain. "My neck, lower back, and left hip ached all the time. My orthopedist referred me to a physical therapist, and that worked for a while, but when I returned to teaching, I was in trouble. I could no longer sit in a warm whirlpool spa all morning—and when I stood to teach, I hurt. A new student teacher was assigned to help me the first week back at school. Twenty-three-year-old Sue Chen was originally from China and had come to the United States for college and graduate school. Hearing about my accident and resulting injuries, she told me about acupressure and the principles behind it. Sue said it had helped her overcome bouts of insomnia when she was under great stress.

"I listened to Sue but was not convinced. How could pressing one point on the body give pain relief somewhere else?

"A few weeks later, the constant pain was wearing on my nerves. I was exhausted from the lack of sleep and overly reactive toward students for no reason; my heart wasn't in teaching. I knew I needed help, but when I took the pain pills the doctor gave me, I couldn't even wake up the next day.

"One afternoon after my students had left the building, Sue saw me rub the back of my neck. She asked if I was having more pain, and I said yes. I had tears running down my cheeks, and I wondered how much more I could endure. Sue came to my desk, quietly took my wrist, and pressed firmly with the end of her index finger and thumb on my skin. I was taken aback for a minute, but she assured me this would not hurt. She then proceeded to press several points on my neck and ankles with firm pressure, yet not enough to hurt.

"Sue massaged my shoulders and the back of my neck, then followed with more pressing of points. After fifteen minutes, I was able to lift both arms up and turn my neck from side to side without intense pain. I was shocked but thrilled with the results of Sue's "acupressure" treatment.

"She explained that the acupressure points have two different ways of working. Sue rubbed the back of my neck at the area of pain and said this was a 'local' point [a point in the same area where you feel pain or tension]. Then she said that same point can relieve pain in a distant part of the body and is then a 'trigger' point. This triggering mechanism works through a human electrical channel called a meridian. The meridians are pathways that connect the acupressure points to each other, as well as to the internal organs.

"As a biology teacher, I've always wanted to know the science behind how the body works. Sue suggested that just as blood vessels carry the blood that nourishes the body physically, the meridians are distinct channels that circulate electrical energy throughout the body.

"Knowing that my chronic pain was beyond scientific treatment, I studied the acupressure handbook Sue gave me. Each afternoon, she would tell me which points to press and how they corresponded to parts of my body. Without realizing it, in less than four weeks, I was virtually pain-free during my active day at school. If my hip would hurt, I would use the method of acupressure Sue taught me and press the corresponding points. If my neck hurt, I would self-massage the back of my neck, then press the trigger points for more relief.

"As I was able to move around with pain, Sue showed me several upper-back stretching exercises for my neck pain. I now do these before bed and again when I awaken. Then, after a fifteen-minute warm shower, I am virtually pain-free. Since acupressure,

There is an old Chinese fisherman's remedy of stimulating the acupressure points that control nausea. This ancient method is now available to anyone via wristbands. The wristbands have a plastic peg that presses the points on the inner surfaces of your wrists. These acupressure wristbands are marketed to ease travel or motion sickness and are available at most natural food and drugstores.

the strongest medicine I've taken is ibuprofen (a nonsteroid anti-inflammatory medication that reduces pain and inflammation).

"While acupressure may not help everyone, I am a convert! I'm now taking courses so I can teach others about this ancient healing therapy."

TUINA

What Is It?
Acupressure is the pressing of acupoints, but Tuina (pronounced "twee-nah") uses different strokes that are applied to specific points, muscle groups, and meridians.

Where Did It Come From?
This massagelike healing art dates back to the Shang dynasty of China, 1700 B.C. There is indication that Tuina massage was used to treat diseases in children and digestive complaints in adults.

How Does It Work?
Most practitioners of healing-touch modalities know that the therapeutic value goes far beyond merely rubbing tissue and stimulating the circulation of body fluids. Tuina relies on the physical expression of Qi, or energy flow, from the giver to the re-

ceiver for ultimate healing. To stimulate health, a Tuina practitioner uses:

- Hand techniques to massage the soft tissue of the body
- Acupressure to touch specific points that affect the flow of Qi
- Manipulation techniques to realign the musculoskeletal system

What's It Good For?

Tuina can help you become aware of your own body and what's going on in it—an essential first step in any healing process. While anyone may find great benefit in Tuina, it can help ease symptoms of chronic pain (headaches, "frozen" shoulder, back pain, osteoarthritis, fibromyalgia, repetitive-strain injury, trapped nerves, sports injury); stress (anxiety, depression, insomnia); female problems (PMS, menstrual pain, menopause symptoms).

Where's the Science?

While the research on Tuina is limited, one case study published in the *American Journal of Acupuncture* (1999) reported some success in treating symptoms of primary Parkinson's disease with a combination of Tuina and acupuncture. In the study, a derivative of Tuina, called forceless spontaneous response or FSR, was used and found to give some relief from tremor and rigidity in PD patients. Researchers reported improved balance and circulation, regardless of the stage of the disease, and some patients were able to reduce conventional medication.

Maddie's Surprising Back Pain Cure
Tuina Eased Back Pain and Relaxed Strained Muscles

Thirty-year-old Maddie O'Brien from Brooklyn first heard about Tuina when she was taking yoga; her teacher mentioned he had received his certification to practice this Oriental therapy. "I had never heard of this healing therapy and wanted to see if it would help my lower back pain. My instructor had attended a school that focused on soft-tissue techniques, such as for muscle sprains or joint injuries. But he was also trained in acupressure for pain relief, so he used both modalities.

"At my first session, I wore very loose clothing. The studio had a healing ambience, with aromatherapy candles burning and soft music playing. My instructor greeted me and asked me to lie down on a floor mat, similar to the one I use for yoga. We talked about some health and lifestyle concerns I had, and I told him about an old back injury from skiing that caused me pain almost daily. He explained that while I would probably feel an immediate decrease in pain, there may be a temporary increase in pain as more energy moves through an area that is inflamed or blocked. Once the blockage is cleared, this brief discomfort is typically followed by a significant improvement in symptoms.

"The first session lasted about thirty minutes. Using a combination of firm pressure on trigger points and sweeping but firm massage techniques, he worked on my back to ease the tension and pain. It reminded me of a Swedish massage I'd had on a cruise, but with more of a specific mission—to ease my lower back pain. As he massaged and put pressure on my lower back, he noted how tight it was and said I carried all the worries of my life in that area. I found myself pouring out my life story, particularly the recent death of a childhood friend. Within minutes I was crying uncontrollably, yet my instructor was not alarmed. He listened and calmly continued the firm touch and pressure techniques.

"When he finished the session, I stayed on the mat for about fifteen minutes, feeling a great sense of release from the pent-up emotions I had held inside. The Tuina massage was not relaxing, as some may think, but it did something to help me get in touch with the emotional root of my chronic tension and back pain. When I finally got up to go back to work, I felt so light and energetic. The nagging dull pain that was usually in my back was gone, and I felt younger.

"I continued to go to for Tuina treatments weekly for a few months. Now I go as needed when I feel especially stressed or tense."

ESM USES ACUPRESSURE TO REDUCE EMOTIONAL ILLS

What Is It?

When regular psychotherapy failed to relieve Michael Melton's anger and anxiety, this thirty-five-year-old accountant from Los Angeles turned to a new type of energy psychology called emotional self-management (ESM), developed by Dr. George Pratt and Dr. Peter T. Lambrou, two California-based psychologists who are both on staff at Scripps Memorial Hospital, La Jolla, California, and on the faculty of the University of California at San Diego. Michael learned that this form of thought therapy is based on the principle that negative emotions actually get lodged in the body and can be released—literally—through tapping, a form of acupressure. Through ESM and self-tapping, this young man was able to relieve his anxiety before it interrupted his life.

Where Did It Come From?

ESM is a blend of several healing concepts, including the meridian system of subtle energy in the body, which is the basis of acupuncture and acupressure, and a medical therapy using magnetic or electrical energy fields, such as electroacupuncture, biofeedback, or magnetic field therapy.

How Does It Work?

With ESM, the practitioner teaches the patient how to self-tap on a myriad of points that are known to reduce stress and negative emotion. Dr. Lambrou says that even in their clinical work, the doctors rarely tap on the patient. For small children, the doctors usually instruct the parent to tap on the child's treatment points.

What's It Good For?

Energy medicine is used for a variety of medical problems, such as pain relief, stress reduction, and chronic central nervous-system disorders. The mechanism of the beneficial action is unclear, but the major benefit is lack of toxicity.

Where's the Science?

Experts in energy medicine believe that energy fields produced by the human body may be the most powerful stimulus to healing that is available to us. These field theory scientists explain that touch and pressure affect the body's cells, which alter their charge and subsequently alter the nature of fields generated around these cells, organs, systems, and the entire human structure. These low-level electrical charges can affect large-scale structural changes in the body's fascial net.

In a study reported in *Alternative Therapies in Health Medicine* (1999), researchers sought to assess the fluctuation of extremely high-frequency electromagnetic fields (gamma rays) during treatment and found that healing energy may be more than "subtle," as once thought. In this study, researchers concluded that marked decreases in gamma counts were found at every anatomical site location for all subjects during therapy. This preliminary study may have strong implications for those with cancer, whose survival may be increased because of the radiation hormesis effects of energy therapies.

Face Tapping Helps Three-Year-Old Girl
A Traumatic Procedure Made Easier with ESM

Dr. Lambrou tells of a colleague's daughter who had to undergo a traumatic diagnostic procedure. "The three-year-old girl was suspected of having a kidney problem, and the procedure was to catheterize the child, fill her bladder with saline water, and then empty the bladder while she was being x-rayed. The child had undergone the procedure several months earlier and was hysterical during the twenty-minute procedure and had to be physically restrained by parents, nurses, and technicians. Now the procedure had to be repeated to see if the medications had corrected the problem. That is when the mother called me to ask for help.

"During the radiological procedure, I instructed the parents how and where to tap on their daughter, and we all took turns tapping the little girl at treatment points for anxiety and trauma on the face, upper body, and hands. During the middle of the procedure, the radiologist was called away to an emergency in another x-ray room and the little girl was left catheterized on the steel table with the x-ray emitter above her abdomen.

"For the next fifteen minutes, we continued to treat her with the gentle tapping at points under her eyes, at her collarbone, and on her hands. The child remained calm and without the need for physical restraint. When the radiologist returned and concluded the procedure, the parents were both delighted at the composure of their daughter and at how the method kept her from being retraumatized. As we left the radiology center, the little girl gave me a smile and a hug, the most rewarding payment I could have received."

Post-traumatic Stress Decreased with ESM

A woman was referred to Dr. Pratt, emotional self-management codeveloper, after having been held hostage for ransom for three weeks. "Each day during the ordeal, this woman was threatened with death by drug-crazed men who were seeking money for her return. She managed to escape, and while not physically harmed, she was still a prisoner of her fear that they would find her and harm her. She appeared in the office with her eyes downcast, voice barely audible, and arms wrapped around herself. Now, several months after her escape, she was unable to concentrate to work, was withdrawn from her family and friends, and unable to function in her life.

"As I taught her where to tap on her face, upper body, and hands, and guided her through the technique of emotional release, over the span of forty-five minutes her face relaxed, her body unwound, and the gripping fear was broken. By the next visit she reported that she was getting her life back."

Sigmund Freud Used Touch to Treat Hysteria

Sigmund Freud, an Austrian neurologist and theorist who developed psychoanalysis, had a firm rule on abstinence of touch during therapy. Yet there are reports that even Freud experimented with the use of massage in the treatment of hysteria (a form of mental illness characterized by paralysis without physiologic basis). In 1895 he published a book that explained his methods, entitled *Studies on Hysteria*.

Since that time, there have been exceptions to the rule in psychotherapy that sees physical touch as necessary only when dealing with periods of deep regression, with psychotic anxieties and delusional transference, and with deeply disturbed patients. Psychoanalysts frequently comment that physical contact in the way of handshakes, handholding, hugs, and squeezes on the arm are experienced by both patient and therapist as facilitative.

ACUPUNCTURE: TOUCH WITH NEEDLES

What Is It?

With acupuncture, the practitioner stimulates Qi by inserting needles into meridians, the veinlike routes under the surface of the skin. By twisting the needles, energy blocks are removed and the balance and flow of energy along the pathway are restored.

Where Did It Come From?

Although acupuncture was developed after acupressure, it has been practiced in China for thousands of years. In early times, the Chinese thought disease was closely related to the vascular system, and treatment often involved bleeding with sharp stones. The wind, originally regarded as a demon and an agent of illness, was believed to reside in caves or tunnels. In acupuncture literature, the term for caves is used to designate the holes in the skin through which the Qi flows into and out of the body. Ancient Chinese practitioners thought that by inserting different kinds of needles into these holes, the flow of Qi could be increased or decreased to achieve a more normal state of health.

Acupuncture came to the United States in the late 1800s but has become increasingly popular in the past two decades. At this time, there are more than twenty thousand certified and licensed practitioners, and more than three thousand of these are conventional medical doctors.

How Does It Work?

While experts believe acupuncture works by releasing chemicals in the brain that block pain perception, there are some new studies that suggest peripheral nerve stimulation can modify functional responses within the brain. In this way, the patient's pain tolerance is increased so that one acupuncture treatment may last weeks in helping to alleviate chronic pain.

Every acupuncture treatment begins with four types of examination:

- Asking: The acupuncturist first asks you about your general health.
- Looking: The practitioner will then note your appearance, posture, skin coloration, and tongue.
- Listening: Next he will listen to your breathing patterns, speech, and tone of voice.
- Smelling and touching: The last and most important step of the examination involves touching your skin and taking an accurate pulse.

To receive the treatment, you will lie down on a table or sit in a chair, so the practitioner has access to the skin at specific points. When the tiny needle is inserted into one point on the body, it stimulates nerves in the underlying muscles. According to scientists, this stimulation sends impulses up the spinal cord to the limbic system, a primitive part of the brain. The impulses also go to the midbrain and the pituitary gland. Studies have shown that acupuncture may alter brain chemistry by changing the release of neurotransmitters, biochemical substances that stimulate or inhibit nerve impulses in the brain that relay information about external stimuli and sensations. Studies have also shown that acupuncture affects the parts of the central nervous system related to sensation and involuntary body functions, such as immune reactions and processes whereby your blood pressure, blood flow, and body temperature are regulated.

What's It Good For?

According to a National Institute of Health (NIH) consensus panel of scientists, researchers, and practitioners who convened in November 1997, clinical studies have shown that acupuncture is an effective treatment for nausea caused by surgical anesthesia and cancer chemotherapy, it also soothes dental pain experienced after surgery. The panel found that acupuncture is useful by itself or combined with conventional therapies to treat addiction, headaches, menstrual cramps, tennis elbow, fibromyalgia, myofascial pain, osteoarthritis, lower back pain, carpal tunnel syndrome, and asthma; it can also assist in stroke rehabilitation.

Where's the Science?

There have been a host of physician-led studies on effective acupuncture treatment.

In a recent study published in the *British Medical Journal* (June 2001), researchers at Ludwig-Maximilians University in Germany studied the effect of acupuncture on patients suffering with chronic neck pain, including those who had myofascial pain syndrome lasting more than five years. (Myofascial pain syndrome is muscle pain in specific areas of the neck that may be caused by physical or emotional tension.) Just one week after receiving an acupuncture treatment, more than half of those treated with acupuncture reported greater than 50 percent improvement in pain.

In another small study published in the June 9, 2001, *British Dental Journal*, researchers at King's College in London concluded that acupuncture may help to ease the gag reflex during dental

---

Choosing a Qualified Acupuncturist

Searching the Yellow Pages for a qualified acupuncturist? Write or call the American Academy of Medical Acupuncture (AAMA). This organization, founded in 1987, restricts membership to medical doctors (M.D.'s) and doctors of osteopathy (D.O.'s).

Members have more than 220 hours of formal training and meet the board's stringent requirements. Write to 4929 Wilshire Blvd., Suite 500, Los Angeles, CA, 90036, call 323-937-5514, or check out their website at www.medicalacupuncture.org.

work. In the study, researchers selected ten patients who had to be sedated before any routine dental work or procedures to avoid gagging. Realizing that one of the main nerves involved in swallowing also supplies the part of the ear that houses the antigagging acupuncture point, researchers used ear acupuncture on the study participants. Afterward, all ten patients were able to go through their dental procedures without sedation.

ACUPUNCTURE

Gaining Favor As a Viable Treatment

Acupuncture gained respect and interest in the United States after *New York Times* journalist James Reston visited China with President Richard Nixon and needed an appendectomy. Chinese doctors used acupuncture on Reston both during surgery instead of anesthetics and after surgery, for his postoperative pain control, and his recovery was swift. Curious about this, Reston asked to watch surgery with patients who received only acupuncture for anesthesia. Patients talked with their doctors during the operation and then walked back to their rooms with minimal assistance.

Reston brought acupuncture to the attention of the American public and the scientific community on July 26, 1971, with a front-page article in *The New York Times* that told of his anesthesia-free operation.

WITH THE ASSISTANCE OF 11 OF THE LEADING MEDIAL SPECIALISTS IN PEKING, WHO WERE ASKED BY PREMIER CHOU EN-LAI TO COOPERATE ON THE CASE, PROF. WU WEI-JAN OF THE ANTI-IMPERIALIST HOSPITAL'S SURGICAL STAFF REMOVED MY APPENDIX ON JULY 17 AFTER A NORMAL INJECTION OF [XYLO-CAIN] AND [BENSOCAIN], WHICH ANESTHETIZED THE MIDDLE OF MY BODY. THERE WERE NO COMPLICATIONS, NAUSEA OR VOMITING. I WAS CONSCIOUS THROUGHOUT. . . .

American doctors were stunned by Reston's revealing report. Yet the National Institutes of Health (NIH) took interest in acupuncture for pain relief and began to sponsor physicians' visits to China to learn and investigate acupuncture and its possible effectiveness in Western medicine.

Karen Gets Remarkable Relief
Carpal Tunnel Pain Resolved with Acupuncture

Karen Bateman, a forty-eight-year-old certified massage therapist, evolved into a bodyworker through a personal need to heal her own life, including a need for nurturing and a desire to be happy. "As a woman I suffered common women's ills of migraines, depression, endless life-draining fatigue, and those phantom aches and pains which never show up on X rays. I went to every doctor, took every blood test, tried pills, and tried to squeeze my head into every psychological theory. Nothing worked. My problem was untouched—because I was untouched.

"Postpartum depression hit hard after I gave birth to twin daughters. When my doctor offered me Valium, she triggered the angry determination I needed to find a better way to get strong and happy. A mother of young twins cannot float through life on Valium.

"Then, while still nursing, I developed carpal tunnel syndrome in my left wrist. The doctor gave me pills and cortisone shots, but after nine months and three sets of shots, the problem returned and the doctor told me the next step: surgery. No, I could not do that. My little girls were now running in two different directions, and I needed both hands to grab them out of harm's way.

"I wanted my wrists to heal, to mend, to become strong and whole again, and a friend recommended acupuncture. After only two sessions a week for three months, my wrists were strong. My twins recently turned twenty-one, and I have not had any wrist

[52]

problems since, even though as a bodyworker I get an intense workout almost daily."

Lynn's Amazing Cure from Raynaud's Disease
*"The Pain and Spasms Were Virtually Resolved After Just
a Few Sessions of Acupuncture."*

After exhausting a list of prescription medications without any results, twenty-eight-year-old Lynn found that acupuncture helped to control her symptoms of Raynaud's disease, a vascular disorder that affects many, particularly women.

With Raynaud's disease, the small arteries of the hands and, less commonly, the feet begin to spasm during exposure to cold or stress. Lynn's fingers would appear almost white if she went out without heavy gloves when the temperatures were cold. If she was under great stress, such as when her father was ill, her hands and feet would feel icy cold all the time. "Sometimes my fingers would throb because of the lack of blood flow," Lynn said.

"The rheumatologist I was seeing finally tried me on a heart medication that dilates the small arteries. While the medication worked to resolve my pain, the side effects were just not acceptable to me. Then my doctor said to avoid cold weather, iced drinks, and washing my hands. Well, that wasn't possible, either!

"My medical doctor is the one who finally suggested acupuncture. She had read some preliminary studies from Germany, and the results, while not conclusive, seemed promising.

"I saw the acupuncture doctor, who was also a medical doctor, for ten visits. At each visit, she carefully placed needles in various points and left these in place for about fifteen minutes. Sometimes she would twist the needles to get better results.

"At visits one, five, and ten, she exposed my hands to cold air from a refrigerator. Of course, on week one, my fingers immediately started to sting and feel icy. The pain was excruciating. Yet this reaction was less on week five. On week ten, my fingers felt a little cold, but it was not horrible. There was no numbing pain or throbbing. I was quite pleased!

"I continued to see the acupuncturist for five more visits, then saw her once a month for six months. The treatment kept my hands at the same level as on session ten—with no pain or throbbing."

New Hope for Drug Dependency

For those who are drug- or alcohol-dependent, acupuncture may give hope for a "cure." In the early seventies, a Hong Kong neurosurgeon, H. L. Wen, M.D., was experimenting to see if preoperative acupuncture could be used in lieu of surgical anesthesia. When he used the needle therapy to treat postoperative pain in a man who was also withdrawing from heroin, he noticed that the patient's withdrawal symptoms disappeared. Wen went on treating narcotic addictions with acupuncture, and reports of his success reached doctors around the world, including the staff at Lincoln Hospital in New York City, who adopted the approach in the mid-1970s. Since that time, the use of acupuncture has spread to hundreds of drug-rehab programs around the world.

Lincoln Hospital has been treating drug addicts with a combination therapy of acupuncture and counseling; more than 60 percent of patients stay in the acupuncture-rehab program for longer than three months. This is quite a large number, especially considering the relapse rate with drug addiction. Today this program is used as a model in more than four hundred detoxification programs in the United States and Europe.

In a recent study published in the *Archives of Internal Medicine* (August 2000), researchers gave more proof that auricular acupuncture, or inserting acupuncture needles into the ear— when combined with conventional treatments—may help fight cocaine addiction. Arthur Margolin, a research scientist at Yale

University in New Haven, Connecticut, and his colleagues looked at eighty-two cocaine abusers who were also addicted to heroin and were on a methadone maintenance program to treat that addiction. The study subjects were randomly assigned to one of three groups that underwent five treatments a week for eight weeks. One group had auricular acupuncture, which is a widely used treatment for cocaine addiction approved by the National Acupuncture Detoxification Association, in which needles are inserted into various points of the ear. A second control group received acupuncture in areas not commonly used for the treatment of a disorder, and a third control group viewed a relaxing videotape of nature scenes accompanied by soothing music, but had no acupuncture.

Researchers concluded that, of the fifty-two people who completed the treatment, those treated with auricular acupuncture were less likely than people in the control groups to show evidence of cocaine use during the study. During the final week of the study, almost 54 percent of the acupuncture group were able to provide three consecutive cocaine-free urine samples, in contrast to only 24 percent of those in the needle-insertion control group, and less than 10 percent of those in the relaxation control group.

Because cocaine addiction is a multifaceted disorder, researchers concluded that acupuncture should be one part of a multifaceted treatment program that includes psychological treatment.

The most commonly used method of needle acupuncture for dependency, according to the National Acupuncture Detoxification Association (NADA), consists of five points needled in each ear. The practitioner tries to influence various parts of the body with the corresponding points in the ear. These needles are left in for up to an hour. Other points on the body or ear may be added, depending on the practitioner's discretion. The frequency of visits depends on the person and severity of addiction.

Becky's Miraculous Cure
Ear Acupuncture Ends Becky's Alcohol Dependency

When Becky Neimann finally accepted her problem with alcohol, her doctor recommended acupuncture. This thirty-year-old actress from San Francisco, California, had tried three different times to stop her alcohol dependency, even spending three months in a rehabilitation facility with no success. Her doctor told her that a friend of his from medical school was involved in a 1989 study published in the British medical journal *The Lancet*, which had concluded that acupuncture may help alcoholics quit drinking. Knowing that Becky came from a broken home with a strong family history of alcoholism and drug abuse, her doctor felt she would benefit greatly from this alternative touch therapy, owing particularly to the close contact with a caring professional and a nondrug treatment.

Because acupuncture boosts beta-endorphins—brain chemicals that give a calming feeling to the body—it may help her resist drinking when faced with change or stress. (In addition to their other healing qualities, beta-endorphins may affect withdrawal symptoms, lessening the body's craving for alcohol.)

After the first four sessions, Becky had no desire to drink. She continued the treatment, along with cognitive behavior therapy, which combines two very effective kinds of psychotherapy—cognitive therapy and behavior therapy, and said she felt relaxed and at peace with herself for the first time in years. She continues to see the practitioner for treatment and has been sober for more than three years. Because her cravings are gone, she has begun to move forward in her life. She has been able to focus on the rehabilitation part of the program, which include counseling, job training, and setting new life goals.

Colorpuncture is a system of light therapy that uses colored lights applied to acupuncture points in order to bring about the healthy exchange of information between the body and mind energies. As with other traditional Chinese medicine, colorpuncture is based on the premise that the balanced flow of energy through the meridian system is vital to experience good health. In addition to pain relief and boosted immune functioning, colorpuncture treatments unwind ruminating or negative thought patterns that are limiting, help to reduce trauma, and support optimal healing.

SHIATSU TURNS PRESSURE INTO RELIEF

What Is It?

Shiatsu is another type of touch therapy that draws on the notion of Qi, or energy that flows along meridians throughout the body (discussed on page 33). The sessions focus on relieving pain and helping the body rid itself of any toxins before they develop into illness.

Where Did It Come From?

The healing techniques that are fundamental to shiatsu probably originated in ancient China and later came to Japan. The first syllable in shiatsu, *shi*, means "fingers"; the second, *atsu*, indicates pressure. Therefore, shiatsu means "to apply pressure on the body with the fingers." Shiatsu came from *anma*, meaning massage. It was recommended for people living in the center of China, near the Yellow River. In this area, the culture was developed, and people were doing more mental than physical work.

The Japanese took many things from Chinese culture to change and develop, among them *anma* and acupuncture, which they developed into shiatsu. Over the centuries, information that makes up the shiatsu techniques was gathered through trial and error, and shiatsu as we know it today was founded about a hundred years ago.

How Does It Work?

The shiatsu practitioner applies gentle to deep pressure to specific points on the meridians, called *tsubos*. Practitioners may apply pressure to the *tsubos* using their palms, fingers, elbows, knees, and feet, but they work mostly with their thumbs held side by side or, for more concentrated pressure, on top of each other. Generally, the pressure is held for several seconds and is repeated several times before the practitioner moves to another *tsubo*. The pressure may help to stimulate the body's endorphins to produce a tranquilizing effect, or it may help by loosening up muscles and improving blood circulation.

What's It Good For?

Shiatsu is a touch healing system that has developed over centuries. It has been effective in easing headaches, dizziness, ringing in the ears, eye strain, general fatigue, tension and neck ache, low back pain, constipation, numbness of limbs, insomnia, and poor eating habits. In Japan, shiatsu is often used as a preventive measure rather than as a cure for illness. In the West, it is still used mainly for people who have been unwell and cannot seem to improve through conventional therapy.

Where's the Science?

In a timely study published in *Acupuncture and Electrotherapy Research* (1996), researchers concluded that patients with severe angina pectoris, a painful heart condition, may benefit from a combined use of shiatsu, acupuncture, and lifestyle changes. In the study performed at the Acupuncture Center in Klampenborg, Denmark, sixty-nine patients with severe angina pectoris were treated with shiatsu, acupuncture, and lifestyle changes. They were monitored for two years. Of these patients, forty-nine were candidates for coronary-artery bypass grafting (CABG). The remaining twenty patients were rejected from having this heart procedure.

Study results were exciting with the incidence of death and heart attack at 21 percent among the patients undergoing the heart bypass procedure, 15 percent among the patients who had a stent put in, and 7 percent among the patients treated with alternative therapies. In fact, 61 percent of those treated with shiatsu, acupuncture, and lifestyle changes postponed the invasive heart procedure. (All reported about the same pain response.) Researchers concluded that these alternative therapies, including shiatsu, may have value for patients with severe angina.

Richard's Extraordinary New Life
"Shiatsu Transformed My Life from Being a Total Wreck to Excited and Hopeful Again"

When Richard Carter, a forty-three-year-old electrical engineer from Dallas, Texas, saw a shiatsu practitioner, he wore an oversize hat, hoping that no one would recognize him. "When I hit forty, I was a wreck—physically, emotionally, and spiritually. I had an excellent career as an engineer, but after a messy divorce, I was broke, alone, and felt horrible all the time. I lived in a one-bedroom apartment and survived on fast food. I never exercised and had no friends because of the divorce. If you saw me then, you would have thought I was ten years older. You probably wouldn't have liked me much, either, because I didn't like myself."

When Richard first saw Maki Hinata, a shiatsu practitioner, he suffered from a variety of ailments, all stress-related. He had cluster headaches, insomnia, aching muscles, and irritability. He was overweight and sedentary, and because he ached and felt tired, his productivity at work was slowing down. He took Percocet (a narcotic pain pill)—as many as twenty a week—to ease his back pain.

"I was a skeptic about any type of alternative treatment, trust me. I'm an engineer who must be convinced with facts before I believe in something that is not scientifically substantiated. I'd heard about Maki's clinic from some ladies at work. It sounded good to me—that she could help me relax and maybe end some of this pain. The pain medication made me groggy, and that affected my work.

"After having one shiatsu treatment, it became totally clear to me that it was based on the laws of physics. This is the study of motion and reaction produced by external forces. In physics, there is a law that states that when there is a force exerted on one object, there is an equal and opposite force or reaction on a first object by the second. In shiatsu, when stimulation is applied to the body, as either pressing, rubbing, or kneading, the body accordingly produces some internal changes. As my practitioner detected internal reactions, she then applied other stimulation. Thus, a practitioner of these techniques applies dynamic stimulation to the patient. The pressure is administered rhythmically in varying degrees, so that the recipient feels the compound results of varying applications of pressure. The direct administration of pressure in shiatsu is simple and linear."

AYURVEDIC MASSAGE HELPS HEAL AND RELAX

What Is It?

Ayurvedic massage is an ancient Indian therapy that focuses on relaxation, prevention of disease, and treating ailments. Hands-on or touch therapies probably came to India from neighboring China and surrounding countries.

Where Did It Come From?

While most historical records describing touch as medicine were written by physicians, the records of Indian massage focus on its sensual qualities. The five-thousand-year-old Ayurveda, a traditional Indian system of medicine, describes body massage with oil and spices. Sensual massage records descriptions of massage treatments and daily activities at the *tshanpau*, or bath. The erotic sculptures at Khajuraho give witness to a culture that uses massage to arouse and calm people. In fact, in the Kama Sutra, the great Indian saint Vatsayana mentions massage for enhancing vitality and sex between partners.

Because Ayurveda was rooted within the family customs and culture of India, the therapies survived through generations of foreign rulers who tried to impose other, more conventional medical treatments on the people.

When India became independent in 1947, Ayurvedic medicine flourished in popularity. With the help of Maharishi Mahesh Yogi, the founder of transcendental meditation, the therapies were brought to the Western nations and visibility increased.

How Does It Work?

According to Ayurveda, health is the state of balance, and disease is the state of imbalance. Its premise is that the body's functions are composed of combinations of five elements: air, fire, space, water, and earth. There are three other physiological forces called *doshas* (*vata*, *pitta*, and *kapha*) in which the five elements are manifest. All of us are made of a combination of *doshas* that give us a particular metabolic type, yet we each have one dosha that dominates. *Vata* people are thin and energetic, while *pittas* are medium both physically and psychologically and hot-tempered, and *kaphas* are slow and solid.

Ayurvedic massage is said to unblock invisible "marma" points, or those through which energy flows. When this energy is freed, your body will heal itself. Today Abhayanga massage (four-handed or dual massage) is offered at many spas throughout the world. Using a special herbal oil chosen for your particular *dosha*, two therapists massage you at the same time. This intense touch therapy is followed by an energetic rubdown with a coarse towel.

What's It Good For?

Ayurvedic massage is used for a host of stress-related illnesses, to reverse the damage from negative lifestyle habits, and to maintain balance in the body.

Where's the Science?

Herbal therapies are used frequently in Ayurvedic medicine and with promising results. In a study reported in the *Journal of Ethnopharmacology* (1990), researchers set out to see if the herb ginger (*Zingiber officinale*) would give as much pain relief as conventional pharmaceuticals for migraine headache. The most commonly used migraine medications include ergotamine and di-hydroergotamine, iprazochrome, pizotifen, and diazepam; and nonsteroidal anti-inflammatory drugs, such as aspirin, ibuprofen, and paracetamol. Yet all of these drugs have side effects and can't be used safely by everyone with migraines. Ayurvedic medicine recommends ginger for neurological disorders, and researchers in this study concluded that the spicy herb may help to resolve migraine headache pain without any side effects.

Zoe's Astounding Asthma Cure
Ayurvedic Massage Ended a Long Bout with Asthma

Nine-year-old Zoe Michaelson from Atlanta, Georgia, had seen conventional medical doctors all her life, trying to find the right treatment for her allergies and asthma. Yet it wasn't until she was

A Touch of Health

BLISS AT YOUR FINGERTIPS: AYURVEDIC SELF-MASSAGE

How can a ritual so luxuriously relaxing, so blissfully comforting as a full-body warm-oil massage, rev up your body and mind, preparing them for peak performance? Ayurveda, the five-thousand-year-old holistic healing tradition from India, has an explanation for the seeming contradiction. Accumulated stress and toxins in the mind and body dissolve during the daily massage. A daily full-body warm-oil massage therefore acts as a powerful recharger and rejuvenator of mind and body.

Abhyanga, the Ayurvedic oil massage, is an integral part of the daily routine recommended by this healing system for overall health and well-being. Traditional Ayurvedic texts wax eloquent on the benefits: "Give yourself a full-body oil massage on a daily basis. It is nourishing, pacifies *vata* and *kapha*, relieves fatigue, provides stamina, pleasure and perfect sleep, enhances the complexion and the luster of the skin, promotes longevity and nourishes all parts of the body."

Here are the benefits that can be expected from regular performance of this pleasant ritual:

- Increased circulation, especially to nerve endings
- Toning of the muscles and the whole physiology
- Calming of the nerves
- Lubrication of the joints
- Increased mental alertness
- Improved elimination of impurities from the body
- Softer, smoother skin
- Increased levels of stamina through the day
- Better, deeper sleep at night

The Ayurvedic massage is traditionally performed in the morning, before your bath or shower. You can use cured sesame oil, an herbalized massage oil, or an aroma massage oil. Look for pure, high-quality, organic carrier oils, combined with pure essential oils for their exquisite aromas and pure cold-pressed extracts from wild-crafted whole herbs.

If you choose sesame oil, cold-pressed, chemical-free organic will give the best results. To cure or purify the sesame oil, heat the oil to 212 degrees Fahrenheit. Remove from heat once this temperature is reached; cool and store for use as needed. Up to a quart of oil can be cured at a time. (Of course, you should observe safety precautions when curing oil. All oils are highly flammable. Use low heat, and don't leave the oil unattended.) You can also find professionally cured sesame oil at stores that sell Ayurvedic products.

Healing herbs are important in Ayurveda. Herbalized massage oils contain a blend of carefully chosen herbs known for their ability to strengthen the physiology and balance the mind. So the daily massage with an herbalized massage oil has twice the beneficial power. Country Mallow, Winter Cherry, and Sensitive Plant are some Ayurvedic herbs you'll find in herbalized massage oils. Country Mallow is renowned for its nourishing effect on the physiology. Winter Cherry, a powerful adaptogenic, meaning it has the power to work as a biological response modifier, aids the body's natural ability to withstand stress and helps balance the mind and emotions. Sensitive Plant helps nerve regeneration. Aroma massage oils also deliver double the benefit—the healing aromas in the massage-oil blend, if properly chosen, are particularly effective in balancing the mind and emotions, while the act of the massage works on both body and mind.

Ayurveda recommends different base oils and aroma blends depending on what you are attempting to balance. Coconut oil, for example, is a cooling base oil. When combined with a relaxing aroma oil such as lavender, this massage oil will be effective in cooling down the mind, body, and emotions. Sweet Orange or Geranium Rose aroma oils are fragrant and relaxing; Basil or Rosemary are vibrant pick-me-ups. If you have a favorite aroma oil or blend, try making your own aroma massage oil by adding five to ten drops of the essential oil, or blend in four ounces of the base oil. Almond oil, a light olive oil, or jojoba oil can all work as base oils. So how is the massage done? Use comfortably warm massage oil. (Store your massage oil in a plastic flip-top and warm it by holding the container under running hot water for a few minutes.) Dip your fingertips into the warm oil and apply it lightly to the entire body. Wait for four to five minutes to let some of the oil absorb into your skin. Then massage the entire body, applying even pressure with the whole hand—palm and fingers. Apply light pressure on sensitive areas such as the abdomen or the heart. Use more oil and spend more time where nerve endings are concentrated, such as the soles of feet, palms of hands, and along the base of the fingernails. Circular motions over rounded areas such as your head or joints, and straight strokes on straight areas such as your arms and legs, work best. After you're done, relax for ten to fifteen minutes, letting the oil and the massage do their magic. Follow with a relaxing warm bath or shower. If your schedule doesn't allow for a daily massage, try and squeeze it in at least three or four times a week. You'll find it's worth it!

Used with permission from Maharishi Ayurveda Products, Colorado Springs, CO. For more information on Ayurveda, go to www.mapi.com.

treated with Ayurvedic massage that her delicate system normalized and she could breathe without obstruction.

Her mother, Karen, shares:"Almost since birth, Zoe has stayed
sick with asthma, allergies, and sinusitis. Our neighbor, a Hindu
woman who is never ill, suggested that I take Zoe to see her doctor, a medical doctor who studied in India and who also practices
Ayurveda. I was hesitant; anything outside the American Medical
Association norm is uncomfortable for me.

"At our first visit with Dr. Gopal, she examined Zoe to determine her *prakriti*, or particular combination of *doshas*. She examined her pulse, tongue, nails, eyes, face, and posture. Then she
asked a series of questions about Zoe's diet, activity, sleep, and
other lifestyle habits.

"Dr. Gopal said that *kapha* was Zoe's dominant *dosha*. When
she explained that *kapha* types are relaxed, slow-moving, tranquil,
and affectionate, I could not believe that it described Zoe's dispo-
sition. *Kaphas* also are thickset and gain weight easily, need a lot of
sleep and warmth, and are prone to sinus problems, allergies, and
asthma.

"While she didn't say what Zoe was allergic to, Dr. Gopal put
her on a detoxification diet of fresh fruits, vegetables, and fish,
along with some Indian spices. She also gave me some herbal
preparations to use to help balance her system and an Ayurvedic
expectorant, a medication to help liquefy the mucus when she got
sick. The herb *tulsi* is the main ingredient, and it helps to mobilize
mucus in bronchitis and asthma.

"Zoe saw a massage practitioner in Dr. Gopal's clinic who did
Ayurvedic massage using rich oils and sweet-smelling herbs. The
practitioner showed me how to use strong, firm pressure on Zoe's
back and chest to help alleviate the tension and lessen her chest
tightness. I learned to use various oils to reduce tension and
relieve congestion.

"Since our visit, Zoe's life has changed. She has reduced her asthma medications, and instead of puffing on her inhaler all day, she is able to use it morning and night and still have an active childhood. That's all I wanted—for my daughter to have a happy, active childhood."

MIGRATION ACROSS THE GLOBE

Touch as medicine spread across the continents from ancient China and India to ancient Greece, where it was used as a remedy for many ailments, particularly sports-related injuries. From Greece, therapeutic touch was integrated into the Roman culture and then moved on to Persia. At that time, as it is today, the full-body massage became popular to loosen stressed muscles, relax nervous tension, and increase the circulation of the blood. Somehow early civilizations seem to know what we are just now realizing—that human touch is probably one of the most mysterious and remarkable healing modalities we have today.

CHAPTER THREE

From Magnets to Manual Manipulation

NINETY-FIVE PERCENT OF DISEASES ARE CAUSED BY DISPLACED VERTEBRAE;
THE REMAINDER BY LUXATIONS OF OTHER JOINTS.

—D. D. Palmer

To gain more insight on the healing power of touch, we must go to the nineteenth century, when touch was used to manipulate and align the skeleton. This period was well before the introduction of allopathic and pharmaceutical medicine, and mainstream medicine depended on touch therapies to give relief and healing to those who were ill. In fact, between 1813 and 1940, more than six hundred articles on touch as therapy were published in such prestigious medical journals as the *British Medical Journal* and the *Journal of the American Medical Association*.

The nineteenth century was a great age for medical and psychic cults. Manual healing methods were commonly used with the belief that dysfunction of one part of the body would affect the function of another body part. For example, both chiropractic medicine, a drug-free health therapy that depends on adjustments to the spine for prevention and treatment of disease, and osteopathic medicine, a modality that focuses on the body's musculoskeletal system and how it is interconnected, are hands-on healing disciplines that originated in the late nineteenth century. Each of these healing disciplines focuses on preventive care and healing the "whole" person. Though the means are varied, the practitioner or doctor pays considerable attention to healthful lifestyle changes, as well as finding the underlying cause of disease.

OSTEOPATHIC MEDICINE IS HANDS-ON TOUCH

What Is It?

Toward the end of the nineteenth century, another touch modality, osteopathic medicine, began to emerge as a new healing art. Osteopathy, the combination of the Greek words for "bone" (*osteon*) and "suffer" (*pathy*) literally requires the laying on of hands, during which the osteopathic physician performs manual maneuvers and techniques to relieve tight joints and muscles and increase optimal health. Some osteopaths say that they "keep a hand on your shoulder instead of a stethoscope on your chest."

Osteopaths specialize in the body's musculoskeletal system and the belief that disturbances in one part of the body impact another. Traditional osteopathy is a medical philosophy and practice that emphasizes the relation between the body's nerves, muscles, bones and organs, and overall health. Doctors of osteopathy (D.O.'s) base diagnosis and treatment on the premise that the body's systems are interconnected. Diagnosing the connection is often done by moving the hands along the patient's body, feeling the body's living anatomy (its flow of fluids, motion and texture of tissues, and structural makeup) and looking for areas that may feel swollen or tense from chronic pain. Osteopathic physicians believe that a patient's illnesses or physical traumas are written into the body's structure. Using a highly developed sense of touch, the physician may be able to detect physical problems that fail to appear on an X ray or other imaging tool.

Where Did It Come From?

Osteopathy was founded in 1874 by an American named Andrew Taylor Still, the son of a pioneer physician. As a child, Still received an informal education, following his father, a minister and physician, on rounds to small communities in the frontiers of Missouri and Tennessee. He then obtained his medical education at the Kansas City College of Physicians and Surgeons in Missouri.

Like most inventors, Dr. Still took a step back from the way things were being done and saw a better way. The young doctor was passionate about the study of human anatomy and the science of healing. It was his knowledge of these two disciplines that brought him to conclude the human body has much in common with a machine: If it is mechanically sound, it should function well.

Still was a typical frontier physician and did farming, mechanical work, and fought in the Civil War. He faced the big epidemics of cholera, malaria, pneumonia, and smallpox. Yet when spinal meningitis took the lives of three of Dr. Andrew Still's children, he set out to search for a better way to practice medicine.

Still believed that many ills—such as headaches, asthma, and leg cramps—were caused by dislocations of the spine and neck. His radically new system of healing was formulated to support good health, instead of acting as merely a cure to specific diseases, and centered around treating the body by improving its natural functions. Still believed that proper structure of the body's musculoskeletal system could be maintained by occasional manipulation of the soft tissues; this would enable the body to function properly and to resist disease by empowering the immune system. Faced with skepticism, he would talk to anyone who would listen about the value of his methods.

As Still's new medical treatments, including manipulation to correct improper body mechanics, began to show results, more people traveled to seek treatment. Soon osteopathy was the most popular therapy available to patients, and Still opened the American School of Osteopathy.

How Does It Work?

Originally, osteopathic medicine was drugless medicine; today it is a complete system of health care. Osteopathic doctors can prescribe all forms of medication, perform all manners of surgery, and pursue all medical specialties. They are fully trained medical doctors (with additional training in the musculoskeletal system) and work alongside their M.D. colleagues in most hospitals. Osteopathic medicine is governed by the American Osteopathic Association.

What's It Good For?

Unlike a conventional medical doctor, an osteopathic physician may use osteopathic manipulative medicine, a science and art that combines osteopathic philosophy, palpatory diagnostic skills, and osteopathic manipulative treatment, the therapeutic application of manually guided forces by an osteopathic physician to improve physiologic function and support wellness. When properly applied, the combination of treatments is curative for primary muscular and skeletal pain and can decrease symptoms (and possibly decrease the need for medications) in systemic diseases. Because osteopathic is holistic therapy, it treats the whole body, not just the affected part. By so doing, osteopathic manipulative treatment is often successful in reducing symptoms, improving outcomes, lowering direct and indirect costs (such as physician office visits), as well as decreasing the frequency of treatments.

Where's the Science?

Osteopathic manipulative therapy (OMT) gives excellent relief for most causes of pain, including lower back pain. Back pain is considered to be like "the common cold," as it affects 90 percent of men and women at some time in their lifetime. But OMT may give new hope to millions, according to a study released in the

New England Journal of Medicine (1999). In the study, patients with low back pain were treated over a twelve-week period with analgesics, nonsteroidal anti-inflammatory drugs (NSAIDs), such as ibuprofen, TENS (see page 112), physical therapy, hot and cold packs, and OMT. The outcome was surprising, as patients received the same pain relief with OMT that they did with more costly therapies. Researchers concluded that OMT was a viable and cost-effective way to reduce back pain and was easily accessible to most people.

PROBLEMS COMMONLY TREATED WITH OSTEOPATHIC MANIPULATION

Allergies	Edema
Asthma	Groin pain
Back pain	Joint pain
Birth trauma	Pleurisy
Bronchitis	Recurrent sore throat
Cerebral palsy	Respiratory illness
Delayed development	Sinusitis
Digestive disorders	Urinary tract problems
Ear, nose, and throat problems	

THE SEVEN BASIC BELIEFS OF OSTEOPATHY

1. Health is a holistic product of mind, body, and environment.

2. The body's structure and function are linked.

3. If a body part isn't working right, it will eventually become diseased.

4. Blood circulation is essential to healing.

5. The body constantly readjusts itself to balance weak areas with strong ones.

6. The body has an innate ability to heal itself.

7. Prevention is central to health care.

An osteopath's finely honed sense of touch feels the dysfunction in the patient's tissues. Osteopathic physicians are trained to monitor tissue texture, tension, and motion; they believe that the body is innately capable of self-healing, though it must constantly fight physical, emotional, chemical, and nutritional stressors to maintain a state of wellness. They use osteopathic manipulative treatment to relieve muscle pain associated with a disease and to help you recover from illness by promoting blood flow through tissues.

If you have a disease that requires medication or surgery, doctors of osteopath recognize that these are necessary elements of treatment.

Luke's Incredible Sinus Cure
Osteopathic Manipulation Resolved Sinus Pain and Congestion

When nine-year-old Luke Solomon had a cold that would not mend and then developed a headache, fever, and discolored mucus, his mother took him to Dr. Thomas Hered, a doctor of osteopath in family practice. Dr. Hered specialized in cranial osteopathy and examined Luke's sinuses and middle ears. The bones in this area are surrounded by delicate membranes and fluid, which have their own slow, rhythmic motion.

Dr. Hered found that in Luke's case, the movement of the fluid was nearly absent. Using his hands as a diagnostic tool, Dr. Hered felt the abnormalities and could tell that the facial tissues were retaining fluid, making Luke more susceptible to infection. He placed his fingers under the base of Luke's head and over his forehead. Then, carefully manipulating the cranial bones, paying close attention to the bones beneath Luke's ears, Hered worked to decrease the fluid buildup and reestablish normal motion.

After the osteopathic manipulative treatment, Luke could breathe through his nose with reduced nasal congestion. He was put on an antibiotic to treat the infection, a decongestant to help the mucus drain, and an analgesic for fever and pain. He finished his antibiotics in two weeks and had no more congestion or cough.

CHIROPRACTIC: HANDS-ON ADJUSTMENT

What Is It?

Chiropractic is an important component of the United States health-care system and the largest alternative medical profession. This drug-free touch therapy is based on the theory that the body is a self-healing organism. Instead of treating the symptoms, such as lower back pain, doctors of chiropractic administer an adjustment or a specific force in a precise direction to a joint that is fixated, locked up, or not moving properly. The adjustment is different from spinal manipulation: It can be applied only to a vertebral malposition (abnormal position) to improve or correct a subluxation. A vertebral subluxation occurs when one or more of the bones of your spine (vertebrae) move out of position and create pressure on or irritate spinal nerves. Spinal nerves are located between each of the bones in your spine. Pressure or irritation on the nerves interferes with the signals traveling over them and causes them to malfunction. Any joint may be manipulated to mobilize the joint or to put the joint through its range of motion.

Where Did It Come From?

In 1885 a group of magnetic healers passed through the town of Davenport, Iowa, where D. D. Palmer, grocer and fish vendor, was earning his livelihood. These healers treated disease by placing their hands upon the patient and letting curative electromagnetic forces ("animal magnetism") flow from the body of the healer through the body of the patient. In the nineteenth century, there were many such healers. Some recognized them as frauds, yet they had a large following who believed in their healing touch. Using magnetism and "laying on of hands" could be a profitable practice if the practitioner had a charismatic enough personality to attract followers.

Around 1886, Palmer, who had dabbled in osteopathy, phrenology, and spiritualism, felt a strong "call" to heal people. He set up a magnetic-healing clinic in Davonport, Iowa. For nine years Palmer was a healer who "magnetized" his patients. It was this magnetic healing that gave Palmer the theory behind chiropractic: "Chiropractic was not evolved from medicine or any other method, except that of magnetic." Palmer identified the unimpeded flow of energy with health and defined illness as obstruction.

Like other magnetic healers, Palmer believed he belonged to a special group of people whose personal magnetism was so extraordinary that he had the ability to cure diseases. In reality, these healers had formed an unrefined way of performing hypnotism. Palmer was passionate in his belief that a single factor was responsible for all illnesses; if that cause could be found, then there would be a simple, single method for eliminating it, and disease would no longer haunt the human race. Palmer felt that many diseases were associated with derangements of the stomach, kidneys, and other organs.

In the late 1800s, Palmer brought his theory to light, believing he had solved the cause of illness—that 95 percent of all diseases are caused by displaced vertebrae, and the remainder by luxations of other joints. Harvey Lillard, a janitor at Palmer's office, had been deaf for seventeen years and couldn't hear even the ticking of a watch. According to the sworn testimony of B. J. Palmer, son of D. D. Palmer, documented in *State of Wisconsin v. S. R. Jansheski* (December 1910), here is what happened:

HARVEY LILLARD WAS A JANITOR IN THE BUILDING IN WHICH FATHER HAD HIS OFFICE. HARVEY CAME IN ONE DAY, THOROUGHLY DEAF. FATHER ASKED HIM HOW LONG HE HAD BEEN DEAF, AND HE TOLD HIM SEVENTEEN YEARS. FATHER SAID, "HOW DID THIS OCCUR?" HARVEY SAID, "I WAS IN A STOOPED, CRAMPED POSITION AND WHILE IN THAT POSITION I FELT SOMETHING POP AND HEARD IT CRACK IN MY BACK."

FATHER LOOKED HIM OVER, LAID HIM DOWN ON THE COT, AND THERE WAS A GREAT SUBLUXATION [MALADJUSTMENT] ON THE BACK. HARVEY SAID HE WENT DEAF WITHIN TWO MINUTES AFTER THAT POPPING OCCURRED IN THE SPINE, AND HE HAD BEEN DEAF EVER SINCE. FATHER REASONED OUT THE FUNDAMENTAL THOUGHT OF THIS THING, WHICH WAS THAT IF SOMETHING WENT WRONG IN THAT BACK AND CAUSED DEAFNESS, THE REDUCTION OF THAT SUBLUXATION WOULD CURE IT. THAT BUMP WAS ADJUSTED—WAS REDUCED—AND WITHIN TEN MINUTES HARVEY HAD HIS HEARING AND HAS HAD IT EVER SINCE.

D. D. Palmer hung out his shingle and began using his theory of disease along with healing touch to cure people. He believed that chiropractic was the combination of a science (knowledge) with an art (adjusting) to provide optimal healing for most diseases. He realized through trial and error that his spinal adjustments allowed people with all forms of pain and disease to heal and recover. He based his philosophy on the notion that all healing is self-healing, and he was merely removing a blockage of the normal healing process.

In 1896 Palmer founded the Palmer School of Magnetic Cure in Davenport, Iowa. This was changed to the Palmer School of Chiropractic in 1904. The first course was a three-week certifica-

Since the beginning of time, there are records indicating the benefits of spinal corrections. Even Socrates advised, "If you would seek health, look first to the spine."

tion course in chiropractic with no entrance exam. The premise behind chiropractic spread like wildfire across the nation, and other chiropractic schools soon shot up, using combined measures such as massage, colon irrigation, and heat lamps. Palmer's son, B. J., succeeded him in leading this school. The Palmer School went on to become the Palmer Chiropractic College, complete with academic standards.

How Does It Work?

Most chiropractors use one common procedure: the quick but not forceful recoil thrust. This thrust is done while you lie belly-down on the special table. In the rotational thrust, another common procedure, you are positioned so your upper body is twisted counter to the pelvis. With the spine rotated to its normal limit, the chiropractor uses a short, fast thrust to realign the spine.

According to doctors of chiropractic, your nervous system controls all functions in your body. Messages must travel from your brain down your spinal cord, then out to the nerves at particular parts of the body, then back up the spinal cord to the brain. The theory is that abnormal positions of the spinal bones may interfere with these messages and are often the underlying cause of many health problems.

The chiropractic doctor may also recommend a program of rehabilitation to stabilize and reduce joint involvement, rehabilitate muscle ligament tissue, and balance nerve impulses.

What's It Good For?

Chiropractic is successfully used to treat back pain, chronic headaches, neck pain, and pain from musculoskeletal injuries. This holistic hands-on care has also been shown to be effective for fibromyalgia, as it helps improve pain levels and increase cervical and lumbar ranges of motion. Carpal tunnel syndrome and other repetitive-strain injuries also respond well to chiropractic, with increased grip strength and reduction of symptoms.

Many patients find great relief from chiropractic, as the doctor provides explanations and concrete experiences that promote a strong patient-physician bond, a sense of caring, and a restored sense of well-being.

Where's the Science?

Proponents of chiropractic tout numerous benefits, from healing back pain to fewer chronic illnesses. In a study published in the *Journal of Manipulative and Physiological Therapeutics* (June 2000), researchers concluded that chiropractic treatments help reduce the number and severity of migraine headaches. Researchers divided 123 migraine sufferers into two groups; one group received placebo treatment, and the other group received a maximum of sixteen chiropractic spinal-manipulation sessions. At the end of the study, those patients who received chiropractic treatment reported significant improvement in migraine frequency and duration of the headaches, as well as reduced medication consumption.

Anne's Remarkable Back-Pain Cure
"Chiropractic Inspired Me to Take Control of My Health"

Anne Stafford, a thirty-nine-year old attorney from Boston, told of being unable to walk one morning about five years ago. "I'll never forget that day for as long as I live. I had set my alarm early that morning because we had a client breakfast meeting.

"When I put my feet on the floor, I had a searing pain that went from my lower back down past my hip and thigh. I had never felt anything like that before. It was almost like an electric shock. When I sat on my right hip, my thigh and leg hurt so badly, it was unbearable. There was a pinching feeling in my hip, and I could hardly walk. All I could think of was that my active life was over."

After a thorough examination, including X rays, Anne's doctor found an inflammation in the spine, possibly from a past injury, which was creating pressure on a nerve. This caused the sciatica—or pain, numbness, and tingling—that traveled down Anne's legs.

Anne's doctor suggested that she work on losing some weight and prescribed regular soaks in moist heat (her backyard Jacuzzi), anti-inflammatory medications, and back-strengthening exercises. She recommended that Anne try chiropractic after a few months.

The chiropractic physician reviewed Anne's medical charts and was reluctant to do spinal manipulation until after the inflammation was gone. He suggested that Anne stay on her prescribed medication and exercise program until she was pain-free, then come back for rehabilitative treatment. He also gave her a weight-loss diet, and some stretching exercises to help increase her range of motion.

Anne wanted to get well. With the lower back pain, she was limited in what she could do—and an attorney who is limited loses clients. After three months, Anne met with her chiropractic doctor again; this time she was experiencing very little pain. After a series of X rays, the doctor felt she could benefit greatly from spinal adjustment; her body was out of alignment from years of poor posture and neglect.

Anne went through eight treatments with the doctor and said

she never felt better in her life. Her posture was better, which alleviated the tiny aches and pains she had felt long before the back problem. After nine months, Anne had lost weight, stood taller, and had more energy. Not only did chiropractic blend with her conventional medical therapy to make her well, but she was inspired to take charge of her health and make positive lifestyle changes.

CHAPTER FOUR

Bodywork, Massage, and New Age Trends

THE DOCTOR OF THE FUTURE WILL GIVE NO MEDICINE BUT WILL INTEREST HIS PATIENT IN THE CARE OF THE HUMAN FRAME, IN DIET, AND IN THE CAUSE AND PREVENTION OF DISEASE.

—Thomas Edison

The first time I met Elizabeth Brock was on a hot summer day in the suburbs of Atlanta, Georgia. I was waiting in line to pay for some organic vegetables and overheard her telling the clerk at a natural-foods store how massage therapy had resolved her problem with high blood pressure. Looking for healing-touch stories, I was intrigued by Elizabeth's experience and began to listen. The forty-seven-year-old mother of three teens said she had been diagnosed with moderate hypertension. Yet instead of going on blood pressure medications, she wanted to first try natural solutions. "My doctor was leery and warned me of the dangers of hypertension," she said, "but I wanted to get my negative-lifestyle issues resolved to see if this made a difference. We agreed that if my blood pressure was still high in three months, I'd start the standard blood pressure medication."

At that time of the diagnosis, Elizabeth was about twenty pounds overweight, hated to exercise, and had been under tremendous stress, dealing with active teenagers while caring for her ill parents. She believed that the combination had resulted in her moderately high blood pressure. This determined woman undertook a complete lifestyle reversal, counting calories and fat grams, reducing sodium in her diet, exercising thirty to forty-five minutes each day, organizing her day so she was not overextended, and committing to a twice-weekly thirty-minute massage. The experimental-massage group was part of a clinical study on hypertension conducted at a local university's medical school. Along with ten other women ages forty-five to fifty-five with hypertension, Elizabeth was assessed on her stress and anxiety level, and then massaged in various positions by bodywork therapists.

"The therapists basically focused on Swedish massage, using different types of strokes, including squeezing, pressing, and pulling motions. For part of the massage, I was in a prone position, and the therapist would massage the back of my legs, my back, and my shoulders and arms. We also were taught various relaxation exercises to do at home, including meditation, deep abdominal breathing, and progressive muscle relaxation. With this technique, you contract and release every muscle in your body, from your forehead to your toes, to try to reduce stress. We did the relaxation exercises on the days we did not have the massages."

Within three months, Elizabeth and her doctor were stunned by the results. She had lost twelve pounds, had much more energy, and her blood pressure was in a normal range for her age. She found that her stress level, which had been extremely high, was greatly reduced, and she did not feel as anxious or nervous. When she did begin to feel overwhelmed, she immediately started her relaxation exercises to gain control of the stress symptoms before they created a health problem.

HOW DOES MASSAGE DE-STRESS?

How did something as simple as massage, along with lifestyle changes, help Elizabeth learn to relax? Some researchers believe that oxytocin gets a boost after a massage. Oxytocin is the hormone best known for its role in inducing labor in childbirth and is tagged the "quintessential maternal hormone." When it is released into the brain, it is known to promote calming and positive social behaviors. In humans, oxytocin stimulates milk ejection during lactation, uterine contraction during birth, and is released during sexual orgasm in both men and women. Some newer studies show that increased levels of oxytocin can also reduce levels of the stress hormone cortisol, ease anxiety, and positively affect relationships.

In a revealing study published in the journal *Psychiatry*, (Summer, 1999) researchers measured oxytocin levels in twenty-five women. They found that blood levels of oxytocin rose significantly following neck and shoulder massages. Because chronic elevation of cortisol is a predictor for early onset of hypertension and other chronic diseases, reducing it may help you live longer and feel healthier.

Rudy's Remarkable Healing
"Massage Therapy Helped Me Stay Healthy Even with HIV"

I met Rudy Pugh, a thirty-nine-year-old software developer, in my dentist's office. When I sat in the chair next to him in the waiting room, I noticed that he was reading a book on bodywork. Curious, I asked him if he believed in the healing power of touch. The young man turned to me and said massage therapy had virtually given him his life back.

Rudy explained that he was HIV-positive. "When the doctor told me that, I wanted to go home and write my obituary because I knew what was next—and it was not pretty."

After getting the HIV diagnosis, Rudy became highly anxious. He stopped seeing his family and friends, took time off from his job, and waited to die. His doctor gave him prescriptions for medications that might help to keep his body from developing full-blown AIDS, but Rudy hated depending solely on pharmaceuticals. Some friends suggested that he turn to holistic therapies to help boost his immune function. He researched diet and illness, the impact of exercise on immune function, and natural ways to destress to keep your body healthy. Rudy said since that time eight years ago, he had become a vegetarian, exercised regularly, practiced yoga twice a day, and was a firm believer in massage therapy. "Of all the lifestyle changes, I know it is the massage therapy keeping me in optimal health. I started out getting a massage three times a week. As I began to feel healthier and more positive about life, I cut back to twice-a-week massages. On days when I feel more anxious, I do self-massage on my body to alleviate the tension. The hands-on therapy has helped me get in touch with my body and how I must take care of it. I now recognize symptoms of illness and treat these early."

Rudy's holistic therapies must work: He had not missed one day of work for more than five years. He said his anxiety level was low, he was no longer depressed, and he hoped to be healthy enough to take advantage of the first AIDS cure when it becomes available.

In a comprehensive study on HIV-positive adults published in the *International Journal of Neuroscience* (February 1996), researchers examined massage-therapy effects on anxiety and depression levels and on immune function. The subjects received a forty-five-minute massage five times weekly for a month. They found that anxiety, stress, and cortisol levels were significantly reduced, and natural killer cells and natural killer cell activity increased, which suggested positive effects on the immune system.

Massage Touches Hearts

After finding relief for a repetitive-stress injury with massage therapy, thirty-seven-year-old Hillary Nelson, a licensed massage therapist, found that bodywork became an integral part of her spiritual path. "I learned to see into the body, to see and feel the blocks, feel the sorrow, and sense the confusion or anger my clients held in their bodies. I learned to listen to the body and, in turn, gently teach my clients how to hear the truths their bodies were revealing.

"In 1995 a friend and I introduced an eight-week massage program for addict mothers and their babies in a long-term drug-rehabilitation residence in Seattle. Carmen had been there for three months with her five-month-old daughter, Maria, who was a crack baby, weighing less than four pounds at birth. She had been kept in the hospital for a month after birth before the court gave her to her mother with the condition that Carmen enter the rehabilitation program and stay drug-free. Carmen and the other mothers received a weekly massage complete with lavender and orange aromatherapy oils, and we taught them a fifteen-minute self-help massage routine. We also taught them how to massage their babies. Of all the mothers, Carmen was the quiet sulker at first. Her body was wound up so tightly, the extreme fuel of the drug and withdrawal cycle turned her muscles into stone. Carmen couldn't look her baby in the eyes; nor did she look at anyone else. So our first massage was in silence. During the second massage, she ask me to do the 'neck thing' that I had done at the first session. During our fifth session, she started to cry as I gently massaged her neck and upper back. Finally she spoke: 'I really want to take care of my baby. I want her to be okay.'

"All the women wanted to take care of their babies. Massaging the mothers helped the women feel loved and integrated a pattern of healthy touch so they could share it with their babies to create a healthier bond. Thursday evening was the baby-massage class, but I soon learned that the babies were getting massaged every night.

"After the experimental program ended and the funding ceased, I never heard what happened to those fragile families. But while we were there, our hands touched the hearts of mothers who could barely afford to feel anything, and their babies learned to relax into their mother's arms. The unfolding of what is best in human beings is what amazes me the most about the power of touch. The stresses of our lives force us underground. Our bodies become the armor we wear in defense against the world, instead of the vehicles through which we enjoy and embrace the world. When we are tense, we cannot know our own desires. We click into automatic and live out of touch with our true nature."

A NEW REVIVAL FOR TOUCH THERAPIES

How can something as simple as human touch give hope and healing to so many? No one really knows the answer to that centuries-old question, for human touch is more complex than any medical instrument or technological invention.

I've described much of the documented history of touch, from the beginning of time to the twentieth century. But in the early 1900s, medicine became more influenced by technology, and physicians who used to focus on touch therapies turned these duties over to nurses and assistants. Doctors wanted to focus more on diagnosis and treatment, using the myriad of new discoveries in the biomedical field.

In the 1930s and '40s, nurses and physical therapists lost interest in massage therapy, virtually abandoning it. With the advent of new pharmaceuticals, such as penicillin, holistic therapies were unheard of, as people wanted a magic pill to cure their ailments. It was in the 1960s and '70s, when the war in Vietnam gave insight into Asian culture, including medical therapies, that a new surge of interest in massage therapy revitalized the field. Some of the new massage techniques were native to cultures around the world but had never been seen before in the West. For example, the forms of massage that come from Asia are based on concepts of anatomy, physiology, and diagnosis that greatly differ from Western concepts.

TRADITIONAL WESTERN MASSAGE

Bodywork (also called manual healing therapy) is the umbrella term that refers to a variety of body manipulation therapies used for relaxation and pain relief. Bodywork includes a myriad of hands-on approaches to working with the body, but massage therapy—the scientific manipulation of the body's soft tissues to normalize those tissues—is perhaps the most popular.

What Is It?

The basic goal of massage therapy is to help the body to heal itself and thereby increase health and well-being. The fundamental medium of massage therapy is human touch. While the various massage methods are described as a series of special techniques, touch is not used solely in a mechanistic way. There is a great artistic component in various manual techniques—gliding, rubbing, kneading, tapping, manipulating, holding, friction pressure, taping, and vibrating—using primarily the hands. Sometimes massage therapists use forearms, elbows, or even their feet to help normalize the body. These techniques affect the musculoskeletal, circulatory-lymphatic, nervous, and other systems of the body.

Leaning on Intuition and Sensitivity

In order to apply pressure without hurting you, the massage therapist must use touch with sensitivity and determine the optimal amount of pressure for each person. This sensitivity or intuition enables the therapist to learn all about your body and specific needs, such as assessing muscle tension, trigger points, or soft-tissue problems.

In the *Subtle Energies and Energy Medicine Journal* (Volume 3, Number 2, 1992), Dr. Daniel Benor describes intuitive diagnosis as a clinical "hunch" that is well known to doctors, nurses, and other health-care professionals. According to Benor, intuition may be as vague as an uneasy feeling that defies laboratory explanation but leads to perseverance until a diagnosis is uncovered. Or it may be an urge to visit a particular patient who turns out to be in urgent need of help. A complex diagnosis may come to mind days before it is confirmed. Occasional intuitive insights are

---

In Touch with Intuition

Dr. Ray Bishop, a certified Rolfer, a system of body education and physical manipulating, tells a story of his second year of practice: "I was working on a female client who had experienced a deep trauma that affected her left side, the specifics of which were unknown to me. During our third session, I noticed a strong smell of burning flesh, yet could see no sign of scarring, and knowing that she had not received radiation therapy, I experienced some confusion. I gently inquired if she had ever been burnt and then described the overpowering smell of burning flesh. After an uncomfortable silence, she began to cry, and as she cried, a flood of disturbing images assaulted me. I saw a large concrete square surrounded in total darkness and a horrific image of a young blond male child chained to the slab, screaming and engulfed in flames. What I eventually learned was that as a child she had witnessed the burning death of a young boy, that she had reached out to him with her left hand, and that the 'deadness' in the left side was a likely result of this trauma. After we discussed this, she began to have increased sensation in her left side, was able to live more comfortably in her body, and, over the next few months, made significant strides in her therapy.

"I had experienced numerous similar experiences and realized that something unusual was transpiring. Somehow I had tapped into a curious world far removed from my traditional academic background and the kinesiological realm of muscular origin, insertion, and action. Also, my whole notion of intuitive sensing and how I could 'read' a body was set on its head. These experiences motivated me to learn more about the science of smell and how others used smell as a diagnostic marker."

reported by scientists, artists, and politicians, and many healers claim that intuitive impressions are a regular aspect of their work.

Sharing Compassion with Touch

Not only does human touch boost physical healing via massage, it is a viable form of intimate communication; sensitive touch can convey a sense of caring. For the bodywork or massage therapist, this communication is an essential element in the therapeutic relationship as the recipient learns to trust the giver. Contradictory to sensitive touch is toxic touch. This type of touch puts the recipient's body on guard, which increases muscle tension.

Elana Dodd, a fifteen-year-veteran massage therapist from Denver, explained that when a massage therapist touches a client's body, she gets an intuitive feeling about the person's innermost needs. "We are taught how to feel the body for weaknesses. From intuitive touch on a massage table, a therapist can tell so many things about how the person is feeling mentally and physically, and often what is going on in his or her personal life."

More Than a Hundred Different Types of Massage or Bodywork

There are more than a hundred different methods classified as massage therapy or bodywork, and approximately sixty of them are under twenty years old. Swedish massage is the most popular, but other types are quickly growing in demand. Techniques used in massage include:

- Effleurage: Gentle stroking along the length of a muscle
- Petrisage: Pressure applied across the width of a muscle
- Friction: Deep massage applied by circular motions of the thumbs or fingertips
- Kneading: Squeezing across the width of a muscle
- Hacking: Light slaps or karate chops

The Root Words of Massage

French	masser	to knead
Greek	massein/masso	to touch, handle, squeeze, or knead
Greek	anatripsis	to rub up
Arabic	mass/mass'h	to press softly
Sanskrit	makeh	to press softly
Chinese	anmo	to press-rub
Chinese	tui-na	to push-pull
Latin	massa	to touch, handle, squeeze, or knead

Where Did It Come From?

Massage dates back for centuries. In the Egyptian tomb of Ankh-mahor, built around 2200 B.C. and known as the Tomb of the Physician, one of the wall paintings depicts two men having their extremities treated with massage. The Roman naturalist Pliny was said to be regularly rubbed to ease his asthma, and Julius Caesar was pinched all over daily to ease headaches and neuralgia.

Massage was not a prominent medical therapy until the early 1800s, when people such as Per Henrik Ling—a physiologist, fencing master, and gymnast—began to study this hands-on therapy. Ling suffered from chronic and painful arthritis and sought a cure. Often referred to as the father of modern massage, Ling even traveled to China to learn the various techniques. On his return, he developed a system of medical gymnastics known as the Swedish movement cure. These techniques included effleurage, or stroking; petrisage, or pressing and squeezing; and tapotement, or stroking. His system of massage was integrated later into Swedish massage. In 1813 Ling formed the Royal Gymnastic Central Institute in Stockholm, Sweden.

By the mid-1880s, Ling's method for healing the body with

touch had spread across the world, particularly in Europe and Russia. People seeking cures for illness came to Germany and France, where many of the massage teaching institutions were located. The "cure" was holistic in philosophy and involved drinking gallons of mineral water, taking mineral baths, doing graduated exercise, and having hands-on massage.

Mathias Roth—one of Ling's most prominent students—was an English physician who published the first English book on the Swedish movement cure in 1851. Roth then inspired New York physician Charles Taylor to learn the massage movements. Taylor subsequently introduced massage to America in 1858. Taylor's brother, George Henry Taylor, attended the massage institute in Stockholm and later wrote *The Swedish Movement Cure*, the first American written book on Swedish massage. After the Civil War, George and Charles opened the first massage-therapy clinic in the United States. In the 1870s, about the time Swedish physicians began opening Swedish movement cure clinics in Washington, D.C., and Boston, the Germans began to combine the Swedish massage with various forms of hydrotherapy. Not to be left out, the English began to develop a hybrid method they call physiotherapy, a method of treatment that encourages health without the use of drugs.

Around 1890, Boston physician Douglas Graham published an article in the *Saint Louis Medical and Surgical Journal* entitled "Recent Developments in the History of Massage: Historical, Physiological, Medical and Surgical." Graham was thought to be the first doctor to use massage as therapy in his medical practice. He helped found the American Physical Education Association and is considered by many to be the father of Swedish massage in the United States.

As medicine became more high-tech in the early 1900s, massage lost popularity. Yet after World War I and II, an interest in massage therapy began to soar as nurses used this natural hands-on treatment to help heal ailing soldiers, following in the compassionate touch-therapy mode taught by Florence Nightingale.

How Does It Work?

Massage stimulates the flow of lymph. This bodily fluid carries wastes and impurities away from tissues and needs muscle contractions to move efficiently through out the body. If you are sedentary, your body may experience stagnant lymph flow. If you are too active, your body may not be able to carry away all the waste that is produced.

With Swedish massage, the practitioner uses a system of long strokes, kneading, and friction to palpitate the more superficial layers of the muscles. This hands-on touch is combined with active and passive movements of the joints, and oil is usually used to facilitate the stroking and kneading of the body, thereby stimulating metabolism and circulation. The therapist applies pressure and rubs the muscles in the same direction as the flow of blood returning to the heart. Swedish massage is said to help flush the tissue of lactic and uric acids and other metabolic wastes, as well as to improve circulation without increasing the load on the heart.

What's It Good For?

The many benefits of Swedish massage include increased relaxation, greater mobility of joints, decreased muscle tightness, and improved circulation, which may speed healing and reduce swelling from injury.

Where's the Science?

Studies at the University of California at Irvine concluded that patients who received a combination of Swedish massage and acupressure prior to chemotherapy experienced less pain and nausea during and after the treatment. Surgical patients who had Swedish

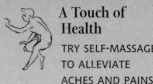

A Touch of Health

TRY SELF-MASSAGE TO ALLEVIATE ACHES AND PAINS

You don't have to get a professional massage to benefit from touch therapy. If you have tension in your neck or shoulders, you can massage these areas gently with your fingers to ease tight muscles and decrease stiffness.

1. Take a few drops of your favorite massage oil (sesame, lavender, patchouli, or lemon) in your hand. With your fingertips, gently touch the back of your neck about two inches below the hairline.
2. As you make contact with the skin, start using a circular motion with your fingertips, moving up and down the neck.
3. Work outward down the side of the neck to your shoulders, continuing the circular motion.
4. Squeeze your shoulders with your opposite hand, one at a time. Then, using long, stroking motions, sweep the skin from the neck to the shoulder and down to the elbow.

massage before the operation required less medication than those who did not. In a study of hospital nurses published in the *Journal of Perianesthesia Nursing* (June 1999), researchers found that after eight fifteen-minute massages, pain and tension were greatly reduced.

In another excellent study published in the *International Journal of Neuroscience* (September 1996) by Dr. Tiffany Fields and other researchers at the University of Miami Touch Institute, massage therapy was found to reduce anxiety and enhance electroencephalography or electrical recording of brain activity (EEG) pattern of alertness and math computations.

Credentials

The Commission on Massage Training Accreditation (COMTA) is one of the main regulatory institutions for the massage-therapy industry. A majority of the U.S. regulates massage therapists and requires five hundred hours of instruction before licensing. A registered massage therapist must hold the appropriate diploma, certificate, or equivalent from an accredited vocational massage-therapy school.

Associated Bodywork and Massage Professionals (ABMP)

provides professional support and legislative advocacy for massage therapists and bodyworkers. Membership is of two levels: The practitioner level requires a hundred hours of training. The professional level requires five hundred hours or state license or registration. ABMP also publishes *Massage & Bodywork* magazine.

Mira's Surprising Cure from Fatigue
A Doctor Finds New Energy After Swedish Massage

No matter how tired you are, you can find energizing benefit with Swedish massage. Dr. Mira Abood, a thirty-five-year-old internist from Raleigh-Durham, North Carolina, remembers the first time she got a massage. As a resident in medical school, Abood stayed exhausted all the time. She worked thirty-six-hour hospital shifts and walked from floor to floor; not only did she lose weight, but her body felt ten years older. "I needed a lift," she said, "so for my thirtieth birthday, my husband gave me a morning at a day spa. The first thing I did was go to the masseur and ask for a Swedish massage. I'd read about it and even studied it in a complementary-medicine class in medical school. Swedish massage is the foundation for the other types of massage, with particular attention paid to the back and chest, using a system of long, gliding strokes, kneading, and friction techniques on the more superficial layers of muscles. It's by far the most popular type of traditional European massage and is commonly used in the United States.

"On that day, I had been on call for thirty-six hours and was totally exhausted when I had the massage. Draped in a long white sheet, I lay prone on the massage table. The therapist poured sweet-smelling sesame oil on my back, arms, and legs, and began to gently rub this into my skin. After the therapist finished the thirty minutes of long, sweeping strokes on my trunk and limbs, I felt a tingling sensation all over. I tried to lift my head up, but it felt as if it were melded to the table. My arms and legs were no better, either; they were virtually immovable! The therapist told me to stay on the table and he'd come back to awaken me later.

"I finally awoke three hours later. I did not realize how exhausted I really was, and I felt alive and energized. My body felt lighter, leaner. I don't know how to describe it—you have to have a massage to know how incredible the results can be."

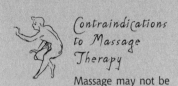

Contraindications to Massage Therapy

Massage may not be indicated in certain cases:
- *Inflammation of the veins*
- *Infectious diseases*
- *Certain types of cancer*
- *Some skin conditions*
- *Certain cardiac problems*

Abby's Easy Childbirth
Perineal Massage Helped a Young Woman in Childbirth

When thirty-one-year-old Abby Cline from New Orleans, Louisiana, was seven months pregnant with her first child, her midwife suggested she start perineal massage to avoid having an episiotomy—an incision near the vagina to ease the delivery of the baby and to lessen tissue tears that occur during childbirth. "My midwife said especially with the first vaginal delivery, perineal massage may help the baby have an easier time and reduce wear and tear on my body."

A perineal massage involves stretching the tissues surrounding the opening to the vagina by inserting a thumb and index finger and gently pulling outward and forward on the lower part of the vagina. This stretching and massage can be done in a warm tub of water, using an oily lubricant to avoid irritation. Women should keep massaging back and forth to increase flexibility in the tissue, which helps to prepare for stretching caused by the baby's head during birth. Abby did the perineal massage until the day she delivered—and with excellent results. She had an easy delivery and did not need an episiotomy. She was pleased, and her doctor intended to share this holistic technique with other pregnant women.

Sports Massage

Sports massage, another form of traditional Western massage, is a therapeutic application of hands-on massage techniques to increase muscle tone and range of motion, and boost blood flow to the site of an injury to promote faster healing.

Neuromuscular Massage Therapy

Another form of traditional Western massage is neuromuscular therapy. It combines the basic principles of Oriental pressure therapies along with a specific hands-on deep-tissue

A Touch of Health
TOUCH RX

If you have a sports injury, remember the R.I.C.E. formula (rest, ice, compress, and elevate).

1. Rest the injured area to prevent fluid from accumulating in the damaged tissue.
2. Ice it as soon as possible to keep inflammation down.
3. Use compression on the injury to limit the spread of swelling.
4. Elevate the injured area. This allows the fluid to drain off the injury by using the force of gravity.

therapy to help reduce chronic muscle or myofascial (soft-tissue) pain. Neuromuscular massage is applied specifically to individual muscles. It is used to increase blood flow, release trigger points (intense knots of muscle tension that refer pain to other parts of the body), and release pressure on nerves caused by soft tissues.

Laura's Extraordinary Healing
Emotional Distress Was Resolved During Neuromuscular Massage

It wasn't until Laura Keller experienced an intense neuromuscular massage that she really understood the depth of its healing power. "I first began to get consistent bodywork from Fred Peters, a teacher who is a very skilled and compassionate neuromuscular therapist (NMT). What I learned about myself from this work was incredible, and I have continued to grow through it.

"I found out that muscles really do hold our emotions. One day my instructor was doing diaphragm work on me due to postural imbalances that he assessed. I was tucked in at the diaphragm, resulting in nasty shoulder pains (computer shoulder), and a forward head posture.

"As Fred did his work, his fingers curled under my rib cage and contracted my rock-hard diaphragm. Fred gently placed one hand on my abdomen as he began the intensive and uncomfortable work on my breathing muscle, and said, 'You hold your grief right here, Laura.'

"The floodgates opened. I wept bitterly, thinking of the recent death of my grandmother and of the tragic loss of my best friend from college. Fred held on to his work, and as I released those tears and allowed the emotions to flow and release, the muscles of my diaphragm also became more normalized.

"Six months later, we were doing diaphragm work in school, and my partner was able to reach four fingers under my ribs, up to her middle knuckle. This is a large and vast improvement. Yet it was not the end to my grieving.

"Fred found more pent-up emotional issues when working on my gluteus (buttocks) that same day. 'I feel your father here,' he said quietly.

"And there were more floods. I began to speak of what made me most angry with my father, and the pain in the area he was working on was intense. Fred finished his treatment, then said, 'Did you feel what was going on in your gluts as you talked about your father? I surely did.' Yes, I admitted that I felt everything. As I felt the anger and frustration, my muscles fired continually and fought the treatment with years of trained defensive contraction."

Manual lymph drainage uses light, rhythmic strokes to improve the flow of lymph, a fluid that circulates throughout the body, carrying away debris and bringing white blood cells to sites of infection. It is used primarily for conditions related to poor lymph flow, including lymphedema (which sometimes afflicts women after a mastectomy), types of edema (swelling), and certain kinds of nerve pain.

Deep-tissue Massage

This type of traditional Western massage is applied with greater pressure and at deeper layers of the muscle than Swedish massage. It releases chronic patterns of muscular tension, using slow strokes, direct pressure, or friction. Often the movements are directed across the grain of the muscles (cross-fiber) with the fingers, thumbs, or elbows.

ROLFING

What Is It?

Rolfing Structural Integration is a technique used to improve posture and body structure by manipulating the body's myofascial (soft-tissue) system.

Where Did It Come From?

Rolfing is named after Dr. Ida P. Rolf, who created a holistic system of soft-tissue manipulation and movement education that organized the whole body in gravity; she eventually named this system Structural Integration.

How Does It Work?
Using their hands, Rolfers manipulate connective tissue, fascial layers, and muscular structures in a carefully orchestrated manner to correct imbalances in the body.

What's It Good For?
The vigorous deep-tissue massage known as Rolfing isn't aimed at any specific injury or ailment. Instead it promises to relieve stress, improve mobility, and boost energy, thus improving your general well-being.

Where's the Science?
Although research is limited, a controlled study conducted by the Department of Kinesiology at University of California at Los Angeles found that people who underwent Rolfing demonstrated a greater range of motion. They were able to move more easily, smoothly, and energetically. Their posture was improved, and they could maintain it more comfortably—in other words, they could stand in a given position without straining themselves to hold it.

Researchers at the University of Maryland obtained similar results. They found that Rolfing resulted in greater physical strength, less stress, and enhanced nervous-system response. This study also noted an improvement in subjects who had curvature of the spine. Children with cerebral palsy benefited from Rolfing, as did people with whiplash and chronic back pain.

Credentials
Training to be a Rolfer can be done at the Rolf Institute of Structural Integration and usually takes about a year for a basic certification. A certified advanced Rolfer is one who has practiced at least five years and has taken an additional six weeks of training.

Julie's Remarkable Cure
Rolfing Helped End Julie's Arthritis Pain

Dancing was Julie Anderson's passion. In fact, this elementary school teacher had taken dancing lessons since she was three years old. As a child and teenager, Julie starred in all the community recitals in her hometown of Newark, New Jersey, then took dance throughout college, and even joined a New York dance company upon graduation. Yet at age forty-five, Julie was feeling the wear and tear on her joints from years of pointe and jazz dancing. She had pain in both hips, which her doctor diagnosed as osteoarthritis, a type of arthritis that commonly affects older adults. In athletes and dancers, osteoarthritis may rear its ugly head at an earlier age. At Julie's last appointment, her rheumatologist said she would probably face a hip replacement as her arthritic condition worsened over the years.

"I certainly did not have time for a hip replacement, and I did not want to deal with weeks of recovery and rehabilitation. I asked a friend about massage therapy to reduce the pain and stiffness, and he told me about John Simon, a Rolfer in our area. Rolfing is a bodywork technique that involves deep manipulation of the fascia to restore the body's natural alignment. The fascia is an interconnected sheet of tissue that surrounds bones, muscles, nerves, and all other internal organs and tissues. Because it runs in one continuous sheet from head to toe, tension in one spot is believed to cause pain in distant muscles, nerves, and more. [Rolfers believe that the fascia toughen and thicken over time, subtly contorting the body and throwing it out of healthy alignment.]

"I consulted with John to see if Rolfing might help my arthritic condition. John gave me a series of ten Rolfing sessions, and then observed that I had an external rotation [turning outward] of the left leg, a rotation of the pelvis, and an unequal distribution of weight on my legs. John said that as a result of my imbalance, the

muscles in my lower back and buttocks were extremely tight to com-
pensate for my pattern of standing,
which put tremendous stress on
my hip joints.

"Using some special Rolfing
techniques, John proceeded to balance my pelvis, bringing my left leg
back into alignment with the hip
joint to allow more proper range of
motion of the joints.

"I noticed that my weight
seemed more properly distributed
over both of my legs, which elim-
inated much of my hip pain. I
also felt more balanced and had
increased flexibility and ease of
movement. Within three months
of the Rolfing sessions, I was asked
to substitute for a dancing teacher
at a local studio. I willingly took on
the task and have never felt better.
I still have a twinge or two from
the osteoarthritis. I know I might
need surgery someday. But for now,
I feel incredible. My body no
longer hurts, and I'm able to be as
active as ever."

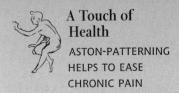

A Touch of Health
ASTON-PATTERNING HELPS TO EASE CHRONIC PAIN

Aston-Patterning, an offshoot
of Rolfing, is a muscle-manip-
ulation system developed by
dancer Judith Aston with the goal
of reeducating muscle movement. Aston combined exercises,
much like an ergonomics lesson,
with a gentler form of Rolfing.
Because it targets chronic muscle
problems, it is highly regarded
by dancers and athletes.

The Aston-Patterning practitioner examines you for muscle
tightness and structural formation, then, depending on the
findings, uses a combination of
massage and education techniques to teach you how to re-
train your muscles. Using a
special "spiraling" technique,
the therapist will work to relax
your muscles and loosen tight
joints, permitting the body to re-
vert to a healthier posture. The
therapist will also teach you special fitness exercises to help keep
muscle patterns healthy, and
will make environmental sugges-
tions, such as changing the
height of your computer chair or
side supports to keep the spine
aligned.

Where's the Science?

The Alexander Technique is commonly used by patients with
chronic back pain. In a study published in the journal *Clinical and
Experimental Rheumatology* (May–June 1996), researchers used a

A Touch of Health

ALEXANDER TECHNIQUE IMPROVES POSTURE AND RESPIRATORY MUSCULAR FUNCTION

There are some reports that the Alexander Technique (AT), a hands-on teaching method that encourages all the body's processes to work more efficiently, may help increase respiratory function. In a study published in the journal *Chest* (August 1992), researchers reported that adults who did proprioceptive (the system that makes us subconsciously aware of where our body and limbs are in space) musculoskeletal education with AT experienced enhanced respiratory muscular function. Adult volunteers in the study were given twenty private AT lessons, including both verbal instruction and hands-on touch therapies, at weekly intervals. Spirometric tests, including maximum static mouth pressures, were assessed before and after each course of lessons. The adults using AT increased length and decreased resting tension of muscles of the torso. This was thought to increase the strength and enhance coordination of the respiratory muscles.

The Alexander Technique is over a century old and teaches clients how to reeducate the mind and body so they are conscious of their movement. F. Matthias Alexander (1869–1955), an Australian actor and vocalist, developed his method of breathing reeducation and psychophysical reeducation from a method of vocal training. His technique deals with the psychophysical coordination of the whole person, as excessive stress in one part of the body is usually part of a larger pattern of habitual malcoordination.

The Alexander Technique helps you to relearn every position you make—from sitting to standing to lying still. The AT practitioner works with you through movement, observing, and patterns of coordination—tension and postural patterns, how you think about moving, and active movement. Because you are an active participant, you will learn to reeducate yourself to effectively change bad habits.

The technique can be very helpful for people dealing with chronic pain, excessive stress, or injury, and is also used at many conservatories to enhance performing techniques.

multidisciplinary approach to treating back pain, with the Alexander Technique as one of the modalities. The other treatments included back anatomy education, psychological intervention, and treatment with acupuncture and chiropractic. At the end of the four-week trial and at a follow-up exam at six months, patients were evaluated as to outcome. The treatment group reported significant improvement in pain rating, pain frequency, and pain medication consumption using the combination therapies. While the Alexander Technique was not an isolated modality, it did help to reduce pain when used in combination with other treatments.

FELDENKRAIS METHOD IMPROVES POSTURE AND FLEXIBILITY

What Is It?

Feldenkrais focuses on improving flexibility, coordination, and range of motion using a hands-on form of kinesthetic communication. Known for its ability to improve posture and flexibility and alleviate muscular tension and pain, this method of moving, sitting, and standing enables your body to work with gravity instead of against it.

Where Did It Come From?

During his time aboard a ship in the British navy, Moshe Feldenkrais developed a chronic knee injury that almost crippled him. When his own doctors couldn't fully restore movement to his injured knee, the Polish physicist and lifelong athlete began synthesizing his knowledge of anatomy, physics, and psychology to develop the Feldenkrais Method. With its emphasis on the importance of making movement a conscious act, the Feldenkrais Method became popular in the seventies.

Credentials

North American Society of Teachers of the Alexander Technique (NASTAT) formed in 1987 to educate the public about the Alexander Technique, to establish and maintain standards for certification of teachers and training courses in the United States, and to ensure that the educational principles of the Alexander Technique are upheld. It publishes a directory of certified teachers. Training to become a teacher takes three years (sixteen hundred hours).

How Does It Work?

The therapist gently guides your limbs through small parts of motions so you can learn to feel the difference between your usual patterns and the new, effortless ones. By helping you to change and expand the way you hold your body and your daily movements, you can gradually reduce the aches and pains experienced from imbalance.

What's It Good For?

Feldenkrais is used for many types of chronic pain, including headache, temporomandibular and other joint disorders, and neck, shoulder, and back pain. It is sometimes used as supportive therapy for people with neuromuscular disorders, such as multiple sclerosis, cerebral palsy, and stroke. Interestingly, the Feldenkrais Method has helped public speakers, dancers, musicians, and politicians get over stage fright.

Where's the Science?

Despite the growing popularity of the Feldenkrais method among touch therapy proponents, there is little research available investigating its efficacy. One revealing study on the therapeutic effects of the Feldenkrais method of awareness through movement was published in *Psychotherapy and Psychosomatic Medical Psychology* (May 1997). In the study, fifteen patients with diagnosed eating disorders who used the Feldenkrais method showed increasing contentment with problematic zones of their body. Patients also reported having more open and self-confident behavior and a better feeling about their health in general.

Credentials

Only people trained by Moshe Feldenkrais or graduates of guild-accredited training programs are eligible to be members of the Feldenkrais Guild. Practitioner members are qualified teachers of Awareness Through Movement and Functional Integration. Associate members are qualified teachers of Awareness Through Movement. The professional training program spans 160 days, over three and a half years.

THE TRAGER METHOD

What Is It?

The Trager approach is a system of movement reeducation or psychophysical integration based on the theory that many physical ailments are caused by patterns of tightness that are held in the unconscious mind as much as in the tissues. Unlike massage, Trager avoids pressure, using gentle, rhythmic rocking and shaking to release tension and loosen joints.

A Touch of Health

MYOFASCIAL RELEASE INTERTWINES WITH PHYSICAL THERAPY

Myofascial release is a way of stretching tissue to make postural and alignment changes by releasing tension in the fascia, or soft tissue. In its natural state, the fascia gives strength and support to the body. But when the fascia becomes constricted due to illness or trauma, it can tighten and pull muscles or bones out of alignment. This form of bodywork is particularly helpful to reduce muscle tension and ease chronic pain.

During a session, the therapist palpates different areas of the body to find the places of restriction. Then, with long strokes, the tissues are gently stretched along the direction of the muscle fibers until the therapist feels resistance. This tension or resistance is held until the soft tissues relax, with the goal of elongating the tissue.

Where Did It Come From?

This touch therapy was developed by Milton Trager, a boxer who later became a physician. When Trager was eighteen, he gave his trainer a massage. The man was greatly impressed, so Trager gave his father, who suffered from tremendous back pain, a similar massage. After two sessions, his father was much better. In the late 1950s, Trager started a practice using his gentle, noninvasive movements to help release deep-seated physical and mental patterns and in turn allow deeper relaxation, increased physical mobility, and better mental clarity.

How Does It Work?
An average Trager session can last from one to one and a half hours. During the session, the practitioner moves the client's trunk and limbs gently and rhythmically so that he or she experiences new freedom of movement. The practitioner's concern is to help the client really feel what relaxation should be like. After the hands-on portion of the session, the therapist gives instruction in the use of Mentastics, a system of movement sequences developed by Trager for the purpose of re-creating and enhancing the sense of lightness and ease of movement initiated on the table. The benefits of the Trager approach are cumulative, though there is no set series of sessions.

What's It Good For?
Trager therapists believe that the deeply relaxed feelings the technique induces can resonate through the nervous system, ultimately benefiting tissues and organs deep within the body.

Where's the Science?
As with many types of massage therapies or bodywork, the scientific substantiation is weak on the Trager approach. At least one clinical study has confirmed that the technique can indeed relieve pain, and another study suggests possible benefits for people with lung problems. However, any other specific therapeutic effects have yet to be verified.

Credentials
Trager therapists train at workshops worldwide in a five-hundred hour certification program.

A FORMER ROLFER FOUNDED HELLERWORK

What Is It?

Hellerwork is a series of eleven one-hour sessions of deep-tissue bodywork and movement education designed to realign the body and release chronic tension and stress. Hellerwork makes the connection between movement and body alignment and restores the body's natural balance from the inside out. Verbal dialogue is used to assist the client in becoming aware of emotional stress that may be related to physical tension.

Where Did It Come From?

Joseph Heller, a Polish born aerospace engineer, became intrigued with physiology and human structure and left engineering to focus on bodywork. He studied with Ida Rolf, the developer of Rolfing, and then, using his background in structural stress, body-energy awareness, and bioenergetics, developed Hellerwork, a new form of bodywork.

How Does It Work?

There are three parts to a Hellerwork session:

1. The structural balance of the body is realized through the systematic release of muscle and connective tissue using a variety of gentle deep-tissue bodywork techniques. This restores the body's optimal natural balance and posture.

2. Movement education is incorporated to enhance fluidity and ease of motion, which helps the client develop a deeper awareness of his or her body and its expression in the world. In Hellerwork, the practitioner will consider how your body is aligned; whether your body's segments are stacked in a straight vertical line from the ground up or are at a tilt or zigzag.

3. The verbal dialogue component of Hellerwork focuses on assisting
   you to become aware of the relationship between your emotions and
   attitudes and your body.

What's It Good For?
Hellerwork offers a conscious approach to changing your body.
Through the dialogue with your practitioner, you learn how to
change negative postures and how to become aware of stored
emotions. Hellerwork is recommended for stress reduction, body
realignment, and optimal health.

Where's the Science?
There are currently no published studies on the benefits of
Hellerwork, although proponents believe it can save hundreds of
dollars in treating and preventing lower back pain.

Credentials
Hellerwork, Inc. training is a 1,250-hour program leading to certification as a Hellerwork practitioner.

THE ROSEN METHOD

Marion Rosen began her career in the 1930s and founded her
training program in 1972. The Rosen method sees the body's ten-
sions as indications of unexpressed feelings or other repressed or
suppressed aspects of the self. The result of such holding patterns,
which may be very subtle, can be lifelong patterns of tension or organic malfunction.

The Rosen method uses gentle, nonintrusive touch and verbal
exchange between practitioner and client to help draw the client's
attention to areas of holding. The technique helps alert the
client to the patterns of tension that are associated with emotional
or unconscious material. This awareness itself is the key that

allows the tension or holding patterns to be released. Often the tightness softens, and the area that was being held begins to move easily with the breath.

Credentials

Certification training for the Rosen Method requires a minimum of five hundred hours of study over a period of four years. Intensive training sessions and a clinical internship are required, and certified practitioners must also hold a state-approved massage certificate.

REFLEXOLOGY

What Is It?

Reflexology, or Zone therapy, is a healing art based on the theory that there are reflex areas, or specific points, in the feet and hands that correspond to all the glands and organs in the body. The term "reflex" refers to the fact that these points are responsive to stimulus.

Where Did It Come From?

While ancient illustrations hint that the early Egyptians, Japanese, and Chinese worked on the feet and hands to promote better

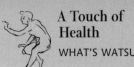

A Touch of Health
WHAT'S WATSU?

Watsu is a type of aquatic bodywork that is used worldwide. Since its discovery fifteen years ago, Watsu has become extremely popular as a form of water massage, as well as a viable therapy for physical, emotional, and spiritual healing.

The Watsu session takes place in chest-high warm water. Working with a practitioner, you receive massage and instruction on flowing, dancelike movements. This serendipitous approach allows the practitioner to use whatever movements emerge in response to the client's immediate needs. You may float in the water horizontally so the spine is freed from the gravitational strain, allowing you to let go of tension and bottled-up emotions that are tightening muscles and joints.

Water dance is a more advanced level of Watsu. With this therapy, the client wears earplugs and is taken through graceful, rocking movements that resemble swimming with dolphins. Water dance is said to be the ultimate in relaxation therapy.

health, it was in the early 1900s that Dr. William Fitzgerald developed Zone therapy, which later became the basis for reflexology as we know it today. In the early 1930s, Eunice Ingham, a physiotherapist, studied the response of different areas of the body to Zone therapy and found that the feet were the most sensitive. Ingham probed the feet, using precise thumb pressure on certain spots, and discovered tender areas. She equated these spots on the feet with the anatomy of the human body.

How Does It Work?
Practitioners believe that nerve pathways exist throughout the body. When any of these pathways is blocked, the body experiences discomfort. Reflexology will help to revive your energy flow and bring your body back into homeostasis, or a state of balance. The Zone-therapy theory, from which reflexology was derived, states that there are ten zones throughout the body—five zones on the right side, five on the left. Reflexes travel through the zones like electrical wiring in your home. These zones are used in determining various locations of reflexes within the hands and feet. All the body parts within any one zone are connected by the nerve pathways and are mirrored in the corresponding reflex zone on the hands and feet.

What's It Good For?
There are different theories regarding the uses of reflexology. Although it is not scientifically proven, some claim that it releases pain-blocking endorphins into the bloodstream. Others say that it relaxes the body and improves circulation. People have experienced relief from allergies, headaches, sinus problems, asthma, backaches, carpal tunnel syndrome, constipation, kidney stones, menstrual distress, prostate problems, and arthritis.

A Touch of Health

Use the following reflex points to see how reflexology corresponds to different body zones.

REFLEX JOINT	CORRESPONDING BODY ZONE
Metatarsal (balls of the feet)	Chest, lung, and shoulder area
Toes	Head and neck
Upper arch	Diaphragm, upper abdominal organs
Lower arch	Pelvic and lower abdominal organs
Heel	Pelvic and sciatic nerve
Outer foot	Arm, shoulder, hip, leg, knee, and lower back
Inner foot	Spine
Ankle area	Reproductive organs and pelvic region

Where's the Science?

Reflexology is now being studied in the alternative-medicine program at New York–Presbyterian Medical Center. Researchers there have found that stimulating a point on the foot can cause a particular part of the brain to light up on a PET scan (Positron Emission Tomography), a computerized tomography machine that shows in color the parts of the brain where nerve cells are working during a certain mental task.

Credentials

The American Academy of Reflexology conducts training in ear, hand, and foot reflexology. The International Institute of Reflexology conducts two-day training sessions nationally and internationally and offers a certification exam in the Ingham method of reflexology.

Ashley's Hay-Fever Cure
Reflexology Ended a College Student's Springtime Hay Fever

"If anyone had told me that having my feet prodded and rubbed would end my annual bout with hay fever, I would have said they were crazy. But it did, and for three years I've had no problems during springtime."

Twenty-two-year-old Ashley Weiss, a senior at the University of Colorado, battled hay fever each spring. She could not remember a time during March, April, and May when she could breathe without taking strong antihistamines or blowing her nose every ten minutes. When she started her undergraduate studies, her bouts of hay fever became more regular. Soon Ashley was having to take medication almost full-time in order to breathe through her nose and avoid congestion.

"One night at the student center, I was talking with some friends about my hay fever. A girl mentioned that she had tried reflexology and it had cleared up her skin problems. She gave me the name of a reflexology practitioner, and I made an appointment the next day.

"The practitioner explained to me that reflexology is based on the principle that there are areas on the feet and hands which correspond to the major glands and organs of the body. By using pressure on a specific area of the foot, an effect will be stimulated on the corresponding area of the body.

"She started massaging my feet and then, using her fingers and thumb, she put pressure on reflex points [also called cuteneo-organ reflex points] to improve the blood supply, to promote the unblocking of nerve impulses, and to help restore homeostasis or balance in my body. After about fifteen minutes, my nose, which had been horribly congested that morning, was completely open. I could breathe without obstruction. I cannot explain how or why it happened, but it was congestion-free.

"As a chemistry major, I'm not one to fall easily for alternative therapies that work without scientific substantiation. But after one session with the reflexology practitioner, I didn't use any antihistamines the rest of that week. My allergist couldn't believe it when I told him! I continued with the sessions for the rest of that quarter and only had to use medication one week when I came down with a cold."

SUPPLEMENTARY TOOLS TO INCREASE HEALING

Hot and Cold Treatments for Relief

In most of the bodywork therapies, practitioners use tools to help boost healing through touch. For example, moist heat is frequently used to help decrease inflammation of a swollen or painful muscle or joint. When used along with deep muscle massage, the technique may offer greater range of motion or increased mobility. Cold therapies, such as ice packs, can reduce muscle spasms that come from joint problems or irritated nerves. Cold is the main treatment for pain caused by inflamed tissues and other swelling. It can stop the urge to scratch an itch and can sometimes relieve pain faster and for a longer time than heat.

Lava Rocks Boost Optimal Healing

Lava stones are now being integrated into some areas of therapeutic massage. Practitioners believe the stones help to turn positive ions (representing congested areas) into negative ions throughout the body. When used with massage therapy, stones help to open and warm the tissues of the skin for optimal healing.

TENS Helps to Control Pain

In some cases of chronic pain, transcutaneous electrical nerve stimulation (TENS) may be used during the massage session. TENS uses electrodes attached by pads to control pain. From 10 to 35 percent of patients with chronic back pain may have increased relief from this therapy.

PERSONALIZE YOUR MASSAGE

While many have tried to limit touch therapy to healing massage, the different types of massage and bodywork are almost limitless—from deep muscle massage to Trager to Watsu to the Alexander Technique. Because each of our bodies is different, our need for touch therapy is also individual. You may benefit from regular tender-point massage to alleviate chronic muscle pain, while your colleague might seek a touch therapy that focuses on posture and movement, such as Feldenkrais. Assess your body's strengths and weaknesses, then review this chapter as you seek the type of touch therapy that is most healing and allows you to feel energized and whole.

CHAPTER FIVE

The Mystery of Faith Healing

THEY SHALL LAY HANDS ON THE SICK, AND THEY SHALL RECOVER.

—Mark 16:18

After Erin Taylor, a young mother from Texas, had surgery for breast cancer, the doctors told her the cancer had spread throughout her body. Six months later, a CAT scan showed no evidence of disease.

When twelve-year-old Kate Bradshaw of New Hampshire was dying of pneumonia after undergoing open heart surgery, doctors told her parents she had less than forty-eight hours to live—yet within twelve hours, her fever was gone. Kate was on the path to full recovery and today has no residual effect from the trauma.

When amateur jockey Randall Scott from Kentucky was in a coma after falling off his horse during a race, his doctors told his wife, "He'll never be the same." Today Randall continues to be a champion jockey.

What do these people have in common? All were healed by faith—the laying on of hands.

FAITH HEALING DEPENDS ON DIVINE INTERVENTION

Miraculous recoveries have been attributed to a myriad of techniques commonly lumped together as faith healing in the name of a greater power. But what is this spiritual side of healing touch? Some claim it is miraculous, yet it's controversial among many. Faith healing is a process through which someone is healed—whether physically, mentally, or spiritually—by what is said to be the direct intervention of divine or supernatural power. Faith healing is unlike conventional medicine, which treats disease with specific therapies developed through observation and research; and is different from alternative medicine, which fights illness with remedies gathered from ancient or traditional lore.

While most Western scientists will tell you faith healing is no substitute for medication or surgery, the belief that prayer, faith, or the divine intervention of a healer can actually cure illness has been present since the beginning of recorded history. The efficacy of faith healing to cure disease has not been scientifically proved, but the popularity and subjective potency of such interventions is indisputable. Although scientists have not been able to measure faith in God or a Higher Power directly, they can measure the impact of faith healing by those who testify to the results.

Victoria's Miraculous Cure
"After Living with Asthma Most of My Life, I Was in Disbelief at This Cure"

Victoria Brooks is a thirty-two-year-old registered nurse from Charleston, South Carolina, who claimed complete recovery from debilitating bronchial asthma as a result of faith healing. She was diagnosed with asthma as a child, and by the time she was out of college, it often took the strongest steroid medications to relieve her bronchial inflammation and subsequent difficulty breathing. "After nursing school, I went on to work at a pediatric hospital, but I had bouts of asthma that put me to bed for weeks at a time. The head nurse was sympathetic to my situation and allowed me time off to recover from each attack or lung infection, but I felt my body declining. I kept waiting for the 'big one' to completely shut down my respiratory function."

Another nurse, Susan, told Victoria about a spiritual healer at a local civic center. While not particularly religious, Victoria was desperate for help with her breathing problems. "Susan and I went together to a faith-healing service, and I sat in the back row, for fear someone I knew would see me. When the spiritual healer asked for requests from the audience, Susan raised her hand and pointed to me.

"The healer and his entourage came down the aisle toward my row. I could feel my throat tightening as people began to stare, probably wondering what could possibly be wrong with such a healthy-looking young woman. The healer motioned for me to come to the center aisle, and I did so reluctantly. I was wheezing softly as I stood before him, and he mumbled something about my respiratory problem. The whole ordeal was worsening my breathing, and I started to go back to my seat when he gently placed his hand on my shoulder and put some sweet-smelling oil on my forehead. My throat began to constrict because of the emotion I felt, and I began to panic, fearing that I would need my inhalers. But the healer did not take his hand off me, and he continued his ceremony. His helpers all joined with their hands, and soon I had ten hands on my head and shoulders while the prayers continued.

"After what seemed an eternity (I was later told it was less than three minutes), the healer told me that I was healed, to go and breathe the fullness of life. I didn't know what he meant. All I knew is I wanted out of there as quickly as possible.

"I grabbed my coat and my friend, and we made a quick exit to our car. Once in the car, I sighed and told her I would literally die if anyone found out we had gone to this place. We drove to a nearby fast-food restaurant to get something to eat. When we got to the restaurant, I realized I'd left my purse in the auditorium—

and in my purse were all my asthma medications. I panicked, yet Susan calmed me down, saying we'd go get it after we ate.

"Then something very interesting happened. In the past when I would get anxious or upset, my bronchial tubes would constrict, and I'd be short of breath and have asthma. This time nothing happened. I was breathing fine. I stared at my stomach as it went up and down with each breath. If you have asthma and typically chest-breathe, you know that is a rare sight!

"I sat down and ate my dinner, then we drove back to the coliseum. The service was over, and Susan and I checked every seat for my purse but didn't find it. After thirty minutes had passed, we gave up and drove home.

"Later that night I was lying in bed, and again I realized I was not wheezing. I wasn't even short of breath—nothing! I was breathing deeply and fully with no restrictions. Exhausted, I fell asleep. At six A.M., I awoke and realized that I didn't use any asthma inhalers the night before. Again I monitored my breathing, and it was regular, deep, and full. The air felt so clean, and I was alert without the normal drowsiness from medications.

"Later that day I mentioned to Susan how I hadn't used medication in more than eighteen hours—something quite rare for me. She smiled knowingly and said, 'What did the healer tell you? Breathe the fullness of life, for you are healed.'

"It's now been four years, and I've used my asthma medications only a few times during the winter cold season. I still see my pulmonologist semiannually, and all my breathing examinations are in the normal range. My doctor still shakes her head when I say I'm virtually asthma-free simply because of a faith healer—but you know what? I am!"

Historical Perspective of Laying On of Hands
It has only been in the past century that medicine became a hands-off practice. The laying on of hands to heal human illness

dates back thousands of years. Its use in ancient Egypt is found in the Ebers papyrus, an ancient Egyptian medical treatise, dated at around 1552 B.C. This document describes the laying on of hands for medical treatment. Before the birth of Jesus Christ, the Greeks used therapeutic touch in their Asklepian temples to heal the sick. The writings of Aristophanes tell of the laying on of hands in Athens to restore a blind man's sight.

Faith healing may occur in relation not only to specially gifted persons but also to specific places. Studies conducted by the medical office of the Catholic church have documented thirty-six "miracles" at Lourdes in which a person was cured of documented disease. Since 1800 a number of Protestant faith-healing groups have appeared, including that of John Alexander Dowie, the Emmanuel movement, and the Peculiar People ("chosen people"), a name applied to numerous Protestant dissenting sects such as the Plumstead peculiars. This group, founded in London in 1838 by John Banyard, refused medical treatment.

There are a host of unorthodox religious groups in America— Seventh-day Adventists, Christian Scientists, Mormons, Jehovah's Witnesses, and Pentecostals—who all have a strong interest in faith healing, including the laying on of hands and healing touch. Ellen Gould White (1827–1915) and Mary Baker Eddy (1821–1910) founded their religious groups around healing experiences. Other women healers, including Maria B. Woodworth-Etter and Aimee Semple McPherson, were instrumental in forming groups of Pentecostals at the turn of the century. Maria was the only leading evangelist of the Holiness Movement who embraced the Pentecostal experience of speaking in tongues. Her healing touch induced a trancelike state in worshipers called "slain in the Spirit," and many who attended Woodworth-Etter's revivals stood for hours having visions, shaking, and rolling on the ground while infused with a Higher Power beyond their physical control. Some even began to speak in a gibberish that would be recognized eighteen years later at the turn-of-the-century Pentecostal outpouring as the baptism of the Holy Ghost.

Based on healing experiences, Mary Caroline ("Myrtle") Fillmore (1845–1931) founded the Unity Church. Fillmore and others communed with the departed by passing hands over the body to unblock vital fluid. These healers are the direct forerunners of New Age trance channeling.

Kathryn Kuhlman is a faith healer who held miracle services from the early 1950s until her death in 1976. Kuhlman had such a strong national following across the nation that she held her famous healing services in Carnegie Hall for twenty years, filling the great auditorium to capacity every time.

Today's Divine Healers

Throughout time, many Protestant ministers, Catholic priests, Jewish rabbis, Islamic imams, and shamans have used the laying on of hands for healing. Today popular televangelists continue to practice spiritual healing with human touch. Evangelist Oral Roberts began his TV career with healing services filmed in the "world's largest gospel tent." Although Roberts does not include faith healing on his television show, he continues to practice the laying on of hands in his crusade meetings around the world.

For Roberts, much of the healing power of God flows through his right hand as a "point of contact." Contributors to the ministry have received the imprint of his hand on a piece of cloth. Oral's son, Richard, now has the gift of healing.

Evangelist Kenneth Copeland is another modern-day faith healer who takes the laying on of hands very seriously. On one of his television broadcasts, Copeland described how he had marched around his home ordering Satan to leave the premises and to "keep off!" Copeland claimed that since then the family's doctor bills have been reduced.

Ernest Angley is perhaps the most flamboyant of modern-day

faith healers. Lines of the afflicted form alongside the stage at his crusade meetings, and Angley attends to them, usually one at a time, laying hands upon their foreheads and proclaiming them healed.

Benny Hinn Ministries report miracles that are truly amazing. After the laying on of hands, one man who had been hit by a train and had pins in his leg was jumping and running all over the platform without any pain; a pregnant woman whose doctors were concerned because her baby had not been moving was overjoyed when she began to feel the kicking of an active child; a nine-year-old boy with a severe visual impairment stated that he could see people, whereas before he saw only dots.

Hugs from Amma

An Indian woman has become known across the globe for miraculous healing simply through hugging others. Amma, also affectionately known in Sanskrit as Ammachi, or "darling mother," was born in 1953 to a destitute fisherman and his wife in a small village in Kerala, in southern India. In her teen years, her love for the Lord surmounted, and she began to attract a following who came to her for love and support.

Called a modern-day saint by many, Amma has toured the world giving out words of love and assurance and warm hugs. In fact, devotees of Mata Amritanandamayi are willing to spend hours in line for just one of her brief hugs. They claim the effect of that one hug—her loving touch—can last them a lifetime.

As Amma greets a follower, she lifts his chin with a finger and dots his forehead with sandalwood paste. Then she wraps her arms around his neck and gently rocks him while rubbing his back and whispering in his ear—"my son," or "my daughter" to a woman—over and over in her native language. The hug lasts about ten seconds, but in a world that is high-tech and low-touch, the hug can feel miraculously therapeutic.

FAITH HEALING TODAY

A number of renowned scientists support the idea of prayer and faith healing. Dr. Larry Dossey, a former chief of staff at Medical City Dallas Hospital and one who has poured more than twenty years of research into prayer-based healing, is a clear-sighted authority on matters concerning prayer and faith. Dossey is the executive editor of *Alternative Therapies in Health and Medicine* and the author of several books about prayer and healing. As a medical doctor trained by conventional Western schools, Dossey called himself an agnostic for a time. Yet he contends that the more he read and inspected, the more impossible he found it to totally ignore the role of prayer in healing the sick.

Where's the Science?

You may wonder how to measure or prove what you cannot see. There are scientists like Dossey who believe faith healing and prayer are directly related to quantum physics, which helps us to understand energy systems and energy fields. Even though we consider ourselves separate entities, the theory of quantum physics dictates that we are inseparable parts of a larger, unified whole. Believers in quantum physics acknowledge that we are all physical beings as well as energetic beings, and we exist as a localized concentration of energy within a vast energy field. You can gain an ability to become "centered," move into an expanded state of consciousness, and intuitively experience the energy field with mind/body exercises such as meditation or ancient disciplines like yoga, t'ai chi, and chi gong.

Rupert Sheldrake, a Cambridge-trained biologist and author of *Dogs That Know When Their Owners Are Coming Home* (Three Rivers, 1998), relates prayer to "morphogenetic fields" unbounded by space or time. Morphogenetic fields are invisibly located in and around organisms and may account for such unexplainable phenomena as the regeneration of severed limbs by worms and salamanders; the sensation of phantom limbs by patients who have suffered the loss of an extremity; the holographic properties of memory and telepathy; and the increasing ease with which new skills are learned as greater quantities of a population acquire them.

Joan Borysenko, Ph.D., a best-selling author, well-known clinical psychologist, and former professor at Harvard Medical School, believes in the theory of nonlocality, which means that your mind can affect other bodies. But conventional Western scientists are stumped when they try to prove nonlocality. Nor can they explain why so many people across the globe truly believe they have experienced extrasensory perception (ESP), near death experiences, or full-scale apparitions of lost loved ones.

So, is faith healing imagined? Is the spiritual power that connects the healer with God or a Higher Power, and also with the patient, caused by a mere delusion or provoked when certain parts of the brain misfire? Harvard's Herbert Benson, M.D., does not think so. Benson, the founding president of the Mind/Body Medical Institute at Beth Israel Deaconess Medical Center in Boston, believes that humans are "wired for God" and, through years of experiments, is trying to scientifically measure the effects of praying for others. Benson posits that religious beliefs should be used in conjunction with modern medicine. He and his colleagues have treated such conditions as hypertension and cardiac arrhythmia with his relaxation response, the common ingredient in his self-care program and prayer/meditation practices. They have successfully treated 75 percent of their insomnia patients, mitigated symptoms of depression in people with AIDS and cancer, and relieved nausea and vomiting related to chemotherapy.

Researcher Daniel Goleman is another believer in "that which you cannot see," maintaining that faith or belief is the hidden ingredient in Western medicine and every traditional system of healing. Doctors have long been aware of its curative power. A large number of illnesses can be treated more successfully if the patient believes in a particular cure. A known example of faith's power over physiological processes is in its influence over blood pressure. According to studies done at the University of Texas Medical Branch in Galveston, devoutly faithful groups of people tend to have lower blood pressure than comparison groups. While there is no proof that faith and belief in God or a Higher Power works to aid in healing, more and more studies show that those who find strength and comfort in their religion have greater survival rates from serious disease.

No matter what is speculated about faith healing and prayer, the proof is not in the science but in the testimony: true stories from those who have experienced healing by faith. A host of researchers are finding increasing evidence that people who consider themselves religious or who feel supported by their community often recover faster from illness than their peers and may even have lower rates of depression, stress, illness, and death. Various studies have linked prayer and religious belief to faster recovery from surgery, substance-abuse prevention and control, and a lower incidence of Alzheimer's disease, as well as a decrease in emphysema, suicide, heart disease, high blood pressure, and cirrhosis of the liver.

Even doctors are getting on the faith-healing bandwagon. A revealing study in the *Journal of the American Medical Association* (May 1998) reported on doctors' renewed interest in spirituality's role in health. One researcher reported that in twenty-two of twenty-seven studies, religious involvement had a positive effect on good health, including cases of cancer. In a massive study published in the *Archives of Internal Medicine* (October 25, 1999), researchers showed that heart patients who had someone praying for them suffered fewer complications than other patients. Whether it's God at work or just a good attitude, patients with rich spiritual lives may have a better chance of recovering from serious illness. In offering explanations, scientists shy away from attributing a supernatural force. But they say that, for certain diseases, religious activity does seem to be associated with better health.

It's important to qualify what is meant by spirituality, for there is a difference between spirituality and religion. Spirituality signifies your search for meaning and connection, particularly your relationship with a Supreme Being—whether God, Allah, Brahman, the Tao, the Absolute, or the Universal Mind. Religion suggests your commitment to an organized set of beliefs and practices endorsed by a community of fellow believers.

How Does It Work?

Clinical psychologist Lawrence LeShan has spent more than forty years working with cancer patients to promote health and healing and has found two main types of mental and spiritual healing methods:

1. TYPE 1 HEALERS: LaShan considers this type to be the most important and prevalent. The healer enters a prayerful, altered state of consciousness in which he views himself and the patient as a single entity. There need be no physical contact, and there is no attempt to do anything or give something to the person in need. Type 1 healers uniformly emphasize the importance of empathy, love, and caring. They state that this type of healing is a natural process that does not violate the laws of innate bodily function but rather speeds up ordinary healing—a very rapid self-repair or self-recuperation.

2. TYPE 2 HEALERS: Type 2 healers do touch the patient and describe some flow of energy through their hands to the patient's area of pathology. Feelings of heat are common in both the patient and the healer.

Laying On of Hands

Janet Morrison has been a faith healer for twenty years. This fifty-seven-year-old ordained pastor from Portland, Oregon, has taught courses in spiritual healing and personally experienced the hands-on healing process three years ago. "For years I have prayed for the sick with laying on of hands and anointing with oil. I believed with all my heart that a power greater than me heard my prayers and intervened with divine healing. Yet when I suffered with a torn rotator cuff after moving into my new home, I was hesitant to let any of my colleagues know about this injury. While I believed that I was a conduit to encourage health and healing among people, I was unsure of the ability of others to do the same for me.

"Finally, when my doctor referred me to a surgeon, I knew I had to try laying on of hands—divine healing—before I went for invasive surgery. The pain in my shoulder was constant, and it was affecting how I slept and how I treated my clients. So after weeks of no relief, I called upon an elder to pray for me.

"The service was in a small chapel outside of Portland, and only a few of my family members and friends attended. The elder lit the candles on the altar, then asked me to come and kneel. Placing his strong hand on my painful shoulder, he prayed aloud to a Higher Power. I could sense the warmth in his fingers, even through my thick sweater. It was as if a magical power was trying to permeate my skin and make its way to the exact place of injury.

"After the elder prayed for about five minutes, one by one, each member of my immediate family and my friends came and knelt beside me, placing their hands on my shoulder while the elder led us in prayer. Following this healing service, my pain had diminished greatly. I was able to continue the anti-inflammatory medications the doctor had prescribed, along with my regular routine of moist-heat applications and exercises to build the range of motion. This was four years ago, and today my shoulder is pain-free."

Janet performs faith healing in several different ways, depending on the person's need and the moment in time. "I do spiritual healing by laying on of hands, when I lightly touch the other person's body. This is usually combined with prayer or chanting of one word, such as 'heal' or 'love.' Sometimes I do faith healing with a specific focused intent and try to visualize the person's problem, whether physical or emotional, and how they are healed of this problem. I often see a shimmery white healing light coming into the wound or into the person's mind. I can use these two processes separately or simultaneously to boost spiritual healing.

"When I do the act of laying on of hands, I fast the entire day and spend much time in prayer. During the ceremony, I say a prayer and ask that the healing energy from a Higher Power (or whatever the person's faith is in) be directed on that person and on her ultimate healing. As I place my hand on the person, I usually feel a sense of energy or tingling flowing from me into the diseased part of the person's body. It's important to understand that it is not I who am healing the person, but rather the energy coming from God or a Higher Power through me into the other person. I am merely a conduit for healing to occur."

While many of the spiritual healings Janet performs could have possible medication explanations, she tells of one healing miracle that was truly miraculous.

A woman had come to see her after consulting with five different doctors about a painful lump in her breast. She had several mammograms, and all five doctors agreed that she probably had breast cancer and needed an immediate biopsy and possible surgery. When the woman came to see Janet, she was severely depressed and almost suicidal.

"I held an immediate healing service for this woman in my

office. I could feel the doubt she had inside, and I felt that if for no other reason, perhaps the laying on of hands would help ease her fears. The woman knelt before me, and I touched the back of her neck and prayed. When I placed my hand on her skin, it was cold and clammy, as if she had no energy or warmth flowing through her body. I pressed firmly into her skin and prayed harder, asking for a divine intervention into this woman's life and the turmoil she was feeling.

"I stopped praying after about fifteen minutes, and the woman remained kneeling in front of me. I quietly observed her in this position, and she was like a child with a soft luminous glow surrounding her. I had never seen anything like that before, and I sat down to catch my breath. The soft light seemed to circle her body, as if divine healing was taking place.

"When the woman stood up, she looked at me, and everything about her was transformed. Her eyes and skin color were glowing, and she seemed to stand taller. She said she knew she didn't have cancer but would proceed with the surgery anyway. She told of having a warm feeling of health and energy almost immediately after undergoing this transformation. The next day she called her doctor and agreed to have the biopsy and surgery, if needed. She was admitted as an outpatient in a local facility and underwent the procedure. When the surgeon called her with the final report, he told her it was not cancer but a blocked milk duct. No further surgery was required, and subsequent tests at six months and a year later revealed no signs of any cancer."

There are other miraculous reports of faith healing with laying on of hands—too many to share in this book. What follows are descriptions of cases reported by other spiritual healers. While the initial goal was to give patients physical and emotional relief during treatment of diseases, the outcome was often surprising:

- Several years ago, Bess, a young mother of three preschoolers, had undergone surgery for cervical cancer. The doctor was considering chemotherapy, as he felt the cancer had spread. Bess wanted to wait until her doctor was certain the chemo was necessary, and she asked a faith healer to treat her. After the healing ceremony and laying on of hands, Bess had another biopsy and abdominal ultrasound. The tests showed that her cervix and uterus were perfectly normal, with no trace of cancer.

- Three years ago, Roger, a fifty-eight-year-old social-services counselor, was diagnosed with prostate cancer. He was told by his urologist that the cancer had metastasized throughout his body and there was virtually no treatment. Even a bone scan and biopsy confirmed the diagnosis. After he underwent three healing services with laying on of hands, Roger's PSA (prostate specific antigen) level had dropped to normal. The urologist did another ultrasound, and though the prostate still appeared larger than normal, the bone scan no longer showed metastases. The counselor told his doctor about the spiritual healing that had taken place, and his doctor didn't believe it was valid. Again, Roger had a laying on of hands, but this time by many of his friends and family members. The next month, his PSA level was still completely normal. Still not convinced that a miracle cure was happening, the urologist wanted more proof and ordered another ultrasound. This time the ultrasound showed the counselor's prostate to be totally normal in size, and to this date he is still in healthy ranges with no residual problems.

- Last year Christie was given the report that she was infertile. After trying to conceive for four years without any results, she and her husband had given up any hope of having a family. Her doctor suggested she try a fertility clinic, using various medications or high-tech artificial reproductive techniques. But Christie wanted to try to conceive naturally. She and her husband went to a healing service they had heard about from a friend at work. During the service, the pastor asked those who were ill to come to the front of the auditorium. Christie and her husband went forward. The pastor prayed for both of them, laid his hands on them, and asked for divine intervention in their fertility problem. Three months later Christie found out she was pregnant.

♦ Five years ago, Juan, a ten-year-old boy from Venezuela, was suffering from muscular dystrophy. He could not walk without a horrible limp, and one of his hands remained tightly fisted. Realizing there was not much that could help him, his mother took him to a healing mass at their Catholic church. It was during the Christmas season, and the church was especially beautiful, with candles and incense burning. The mother and her son sat in the pew, watching the priests and choir lead the congregation in worship. Suddenly, Juan stood up from his seat and began to walk to the altar. The choir continued to sing, and one of the priests met him. The boy asked for healing prayers, and the priest laid his hands on Juan's hand and prayed. Juan remained at the altar for the entire service. His mother said she did not know what he was doing, but after everyone had left, he walked back to his seat to be with her. "He was not limping, and both of his hands were completely opened. I cried as I embraced my son. I didn't understand how this could happen, but we walked home clutching each other."

Later that week, Juan's doctors ran a battery of tests on the young boy and found no sign of MD. To this day, the teenager is able to live a full and active life without disease.

Placebo Effect Is Part of Healing

You may wonder how one knows if faith healing is from God or a Higher Power, or if it just "happened." It's difficult to tell, particularly with the placebo response phenomenon. "Placebo" is Latin for "I shall please" (the opening phrase of the Catholic vespers for the dead, to which the word ironically referred in its original context). Placebos are usually viewed as fake treatments (such as sugar pills) that doctors give merely to calm anxious patients or to indulge insatiable ones. However, it has been shown that the placebo phenomenon yields beneficial effects in 60 to 90 percent of diseases, including angina pectoris, bronchial asthma, herpes simplex, and duodenal ulcer. Three elements are involved in this placebo effect:

1. Positive belief and expectations by the patient

2. Positive belief and expectations by the physician or health-care provider

3. A good relationship between the two parties

Interestingly, some interventions that can be considered placebo, unreal or "fake" therapy, turn out to produce various biochemical or physiologic changes. While not everyone responds to placebos, it is reported that 30 to 40 percent of treated patients do respond to placebo, with up to 55 percent of these patients claiming to have great benefit in terms of pain relief.

BE CAREFUL WHAT YOU ASK FOR

Spiritual Peace for the End of Life's Journey

The laying on of hands is used not only to heal physical or emotional problems; for centuries it has eased the fear of dying for those with terminal illness. Lana Brightman's story is one that has touched the hearts of many. "As a registered nurse in an assisted-living center, it is not unusual for me to treat those with terminal illness. A few years ago, I was called to talk with a sixty-four-year-old woman named Mary who was dying from lymphoma. She had tried to overdose on pain medication while another nurse was on duty. Knowing that I also practiced spiritual healing, the administrator asked me to see if I could ease her fears.

"When I sat down on Mary's bedside, she turned her face from me and asked me to leave, saying she didn't need any witchcraft or hocus-pocus to make her well. I knew she was hardened by the illness and all she was giving up with it—watching her grandchildren grow up and leaving her husband and close friends. But as I touched her icy-cold hands, tears were flowing from her eyes, and she gripped my hands passionately. I sat there clutching her hands, trying to pour out some of the love, health, and warmth from my own body into her frail body.

"As we sat in silence, I noticed pictures of the woman's family on

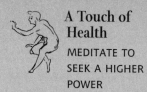

A Touch of Health

MEDITATE TO SEEK A HIGHER POWER

Remember when transcendental meditation was thought to be a cult? Today meditation is recognized as a viable way to lower blood pressure, alleviate insomnia, and reduce chronic pain, as well as get in tune with a Higher Power. This stress releaser seeks to integrate the mind, body, and spirit through intentionally focusing on the silent repetition of a focus word ("love"), sound ("om"), or phrase ("peace heals"). As thoughts intrude, you *mindfully* chant while facilitating the relaxation response.

This technique can guide you beyond the negative thoughts and agitations of the busy mind and allow you to become "unstuck" from your fear and other disturbing emotions. Mindfulness is a traditional Buddhist approach to meditation and allows your mind to be full of whatever you are doing at that moment, whether it is dancing, gardening, writing, or listening to music. Intense focus is the key to mindfulness, as well as the ability to keep negative thoughts from intruding on the moment.

Some people who meditate only occasionally have an opposite reaction, such as increased anxiety or fear during the session. Researchers believe that these feelings may be responses to the sensation of being totally relaxed and uninhibited.

the nightstand next to her bed. I mentioned to her how beautiful her grandchildren were, and she slowly turned to look at the pictures. She listened intently as I talked about experiences with my own four children, including the death of my youngest son to leukemia when he was only five years old. I told her how he was at total peace when he died and how our family had all laid hands on his body, touching him in some way, for about an hour before his death.

"We sat in silence for about twenty minutes, then Mary asked if I'd lay hands on her and pray for strength as she approached death. I quietly complied and placed my hands softly on her skin and prayed aloud. While I was doing this, her husband and two children walked in. Mary's eyes were still closed, and I motioned for them to also place their hands on her body. There we stood around the dying woman, acting as conduits of love and strength. I tiptoed out of the room to give Mary's family a chance to say goodbye. Later that day, a nurse from the floor called me to report Mary's death. She said her family was still surrounding her, touching her in some way, and Mary had a smile upon her face during her last minutes of life."

SEARCHING FOR PROOF

While science searches for proof of faith healing, we are witnesses each day to ways spirituality can heal. Healing is not always about getting well or being healthy. It sometimes means dying with dignity and peace, surrounded by the compassion of those you love.

Today we have entered a new realm of scientific understanding of mechanisms by which faith, belief, and imagination can actually unlock the mysteries of healing. It was two thousand years ago that a woman who had suffered prolonged uterine bleeding approached Jesus of Nazareth. Coming up to him in a crowd, she touched the hem of his garment and was instantly healed. Jesus turned to her and explained that it was her faith that had made her whole.

Perhaps after centuries of trying to make rational explanations of the physical world, even the most dubious scientist can begin to appreciate the truth of this assessment.

CHAPTER SIX

Centering on Therapeutic Touch

TO DO ANY GOOD, THE PUPILS MUST DO EVERYTHING WITH THEIR OWN
HANDS—MUST NOT THEY?

—Florence Nightingale

Ask any nurse or health-care professional about therapeutic touch (TT) and many will have incredible stories to share. Diane, a registered nurse, has used TT on family and friends for more than a decade, finding it to be beneficial for minor "aches and pains." However, when her brother had to have an emergency appendectomy, Diane's healing touch became a most dramatic experience. "My sister-in-law reached me just after my brother was taken into surgery. In fact, I got to the hospital just before he was returned to his room. He was fairly content at the time, but became uncomfortable enough that he decided to put his call-light on to ask for something for pain.

"As we waited for a nurse to appear with pain-relieving medication, my brother became increasingly uncomfortable to the point where he had a fixed furrow between his tightly closed eyes. As a nurse and therapeutic touch practitioner, I had had enough. I started doing therapeutic touch, and as I proceeded in the treatment, my brother's eyelids and furrow relaxed. His body became calm, and he fell into a sleep that brought on snoring. By the time the nurse arrived, my brother had to be awakened and asked if he wanted something for pain. He took a moment to consider and said rather lightheartedly, 'No. I feel pretty good, now.' Of course, I didn't hesitate to tell the nurse that I had done therapeutic touch on him!"

There are many trained scientists and health-care professionals who passionately believe in therapeutic touch, and published journal studies have revealed positive outcomes. For example, in a study published in *Alternative Therapies in Health and Medicine* (March 1997), researchers at Charleston's College of Nursing, Medical University of South Carolina, sought to evaluate the effectiveness of therapeutic touch in reducing the adverse immunological effects of stress in "highly stressed college students." The test group underwent therapeutic-touch sessions, after which the changes in immune function related to anxiety and the relief of anxiety were measured. Researchers concluded that as an intervention, therapeutic touch may be very useful in reducing the adverse immunologic consequences of anxiety related to stress.

Other studies published in prestigious medical journals conclude the same: TT is an extremely useful healing modality.

THERAPEUTIC TOUCH

What Is It?

Therapeutic touch (TT) is a form of compassionate energy-based healing. The trained TT practitioner can sense the human energy field (aura) through hand chakras, or centers of consciousness introduced in Indian mystical writings. These human auras reflect the life force that permeates all things. The term "chakra" is a Sanskrit word meaning "wheel," and it is a concept that comes out of yoga philosophy. In the yoga system, energy is seen as revolving around certain centers located along the spine from the tailbone up to the crown of the head. There are seven chakras, and each one deals with a type of energy in a part of the body.

As proof of the energy field's existence, some cite images of an energy aura taken with Kirilian photography, a technique in which the hands are placed on film and a low-amp electrical current produces a picture that reveals a person's emotional and physical problems before symptoms are felt.

Where Did It Come From?

Therapeutic touch was developed in the early 1970s as a nursing intervention by Dr. Dolores Krieger, a nurse and professor at New York University, along with Dora Kunz, a clairvoyant and healer. TT has been taught at more than a hundred colleges and universities since the 1970s and is currently offered in about seventy health-care facilities nationwide. Krieger has taught the technique to more than fifty thousand health-care professionals and several thousand laypersons.

Biofield Therapeutics

Therapeutic touch is considered a type of biofield therapeutics, which is a very old form of healing. The earliest Eastern references are in the Huang Ti Nei Ching Su Wen (the Yellow Emperor's Classic of Internal Medicine), dated more than five thousand years ago. Practitioners agree that the human biofield permeates the physical body and extends outward for several inches. Extension of the external biofield depends on the person's emotional state and health. Biofield therapeutics works in two ways:

1. The healing force comes from a source other than the practitioner—God, a Higher Power, the cosmos, or another supernatural entity.

2. A human biofield is directed or changed in some way by the practitioner as the operative mechanism.

During biofield treatment, the practitioner places his or her hands directly on or near the patient's body to improve general health or treat a specific dysfunction. Treatment sessions may take from twenty minutes to an hour or more; a series of sessions is often needed to treat some disorders.

How Does It Work?

According to therapeutic touch founder Dr. Dolores Krieger, all the life sciences agree that physically, a human being is an open energy system. In therapeutic touch, one person transfers energy to another. Despite its name, this therapy rarely involves physical contact between the practitioner and patient. Instead, the therapist will move his or her hands just above your body. You'll be asked to sit or lie down before the procedure begins. No disrobing is necessary.

Using the hands to scan the body's energy field (a blueprint that runs through your body and beyond it), TT practitioners look for symmetry, balance, rhythm, and flow. These should be the same on both sides of the body. Practitioners may sense heat, cold, sickness, or heaviness throughout the energy field. Once the assessment is completed, practitioners use this form of touchless healing to rebalance the energy field. This spiritual energy can help speed up the natural healing process of the body and improves recovery time. It can be used to combat serious illness and the effects of treatments such as chemotherapy and radiation therapy.

The phases of TT include:

1. CENTERING: The practitioner uses breath, imagery, meditation, and/or visualizations to bring the body, mind, and emotions to a quiet, focused state of consciousness. Experienced practitioners can usually complete this process within a few minutes.

2. ASSESSING: Holding the hands about two to six inches away from the patient's energy field, the TT practitioner evaluates the condition of the energy field that surrounds the body by moving his or

her hands from the head to the feet in a rhythmical, symmetrical manner. Some experienced practitioners describe feelings of warmth, coolness, static, blockage, pulling, or tingling.

3. INTERVENTION: Also called unruffling, this is done with the hands from the midline of the person while continuing to move from the patient's head to the feet.

4. BALANCING, REBALANCING: In this process, the TT practitioner projects, directs, and modulates the energy based on the nature of the living field, and tries to establish order or balance in the system. When the practitioner finds a "blocked" (congested) area, she moves her hands in a sweeping motion from the top of the location down and away from the body. When a deficit of energy is found, the practitioner will work to transfer energy. If there are areas of congestion, the energy will be repatterned.

5. EVALUATION/CLOSURE: At the end of the treatment, the practitioner will talk to the patient about the experience and invite responses.

What's It Good For?

In early 1994, TT received a research grant awarded to alternative therapies by the U.S. National Institute of Health. Research and experience have shown its effectiveness in:

+ Promotion of relaxation and reduction of anxiety
+ Changing the patient's perception of pain
+ Facilitating the body's natural restorative processes

Lasting about twenty minutes, TT is a process that is always individualized. Some may be more sensitive to TT, including pregnant women, newborns, the elderly or debilitated, the terminally ill, and those with psychiatric or emotional disorders. Although therapeutic touch is used for almost any physical and emotional illnesses, it is best indicated for pain (of all types:

headaches, preoperative and postsurgical, musculoskeletal, neurologic, psychologic); irritability and anxiety; lethargy, fatigue, and depression; PMS; nausea and vomiting; wound healing; chemotherapy and radiation sickness; and hospice.

Where's the Science?

There are studies showing the potential for TT as an effective healing method. One study published in the *Subtle Energies and Energy Medicine Journal* (1990) examined the effect of noncontact therapeutic touch (NCTT) on the rate of surgical wound healing in a double-blind study. Full-thickness dermal wounds were incised on the lateral deltoid region using a skin-punch biopsy instrument on healthy subjects randomly assigned to treatment or control groups. Subjects were blinded both to group assignment and to the true nature of the active treatment modality in order to control placebo and expectation effects. Incisions were dressed with gas-permeable dressings, and wound surface areas were measured on days zero, eight, and sixteen. Active and control treatments were comprised of daily sessions of five minutes of exposure to a hidden therapeutic-touch practitioner or to sham exposure. Results showed that treated subjects experienced a significant acceleration in the rate of wound healing as compared to nontreated subjects.

Credentials

Nurse Healers–Professional Associates International provides information about therapeutic touch and training for health-care providers. The length of training varies, and there is no formal certification.

Healed by a Nurse's Touch

The field of nursing is based on compassionate touch. Florence Nightingale, the founder of modern nursing, believed in hands-on care and used touch to comfort injured soldiers during the war. In 1941 Dr. F. Talbot coined the acronym TLC (tender loving care) after his observation of a grandmotherly hospital volunteer whose loving and cuddling of failure-to-thrive infants miraculously turned them around.

Therapeutic touch is a derivative of the biblical laying on of hands, although it is not done in a religious context, and most of the time it is touchless. Operating on the concept that each person has an energy field that extends beyond his or her physical boundaries, TT practitioners modify or change this energy by passing their hands over the body.

Truth Is Proof

When citing the efficacy of TT, one registered nurse from the Midwest commented that until we find a way to measure each patient's energy field, it will be difficult to show the science behind therapeutic touch.

"What should we say? Oh, Mr. Smith's energy field has dipped ten milligraus since he received his TT treatment. He can be released now; he's healed!

"While science has been able to create devices like an ECG to measure the electricity in the heart, an EEG to measure the electricity in the brain, and even galvanized skin tests to measure the perspiration and response to stress, nobody can measure the energy field quite yet.

"The main thing TT practioners go by is the end result after a treatment. Is the patient improved? Of course there can be a placebo effect between practitioner and patient, as with any treatment intervention, including the most expensive pharmaceutical. However, we've seen people finally find relief from chronic pain, be able to get a good night's sleep, or be free from anxiety prior to surgery and heal faster after surgery. TT practitioners can measure blood pressure before and after TT and see a positive response; that's a measure. We take pulses; we monitor breathing; and we oversee requests for pain medication. We run heart tapes at the nurses' station before and after TT. All of these are scientific medical measurements, and all are used to offer proof to the medical field.

"That's what I learned from Dr. Dolores Krieger. As a nurse, she did what it took to offer a scientific basis for TT. It has been used in very controlled hospital settings in multiple studies and with consistent results. Therapeutic touch is a gentle, subtle healing technique that anyone can learn to do."

Ted's Incredible Healing
"I Was Thrilled by the Results of TT on My Damaged Skin After Radiation Treatments"

Ted leaned on TT when he underwent radiation treatments for prostate cancer. This forty-nine-year-old attorney from Fort Wayne, Indiana, was diagnosed with prostate cancer at a young age. After he underwent surgery, his oncologist recommended radiation to prevent any of the cancer from returning. "I began to experience some skin reactions to the radiation treatment, and the treated areas were turning pink in color, as if the beginning of a burn was starting. While the first two TT sessions were basically uneventful, I suddenly began to feel as if a cool mountain stream was pouring over my treatment area. The therapist asked me what I was feeling, and I described the cool stream coating my parched skin. She said that was exactly what she was visualizing!

"When I arrived home, imagine how amazed I was when all of the pink color was gone and my skin was completely normal in appearance. This occurred in a period of one hour. If this had not happened to me, I may not have believed such dramatic results could occur.

"We continued to meet regularly for ongoing treatments until the middle of June. Then my therapist had to go out of town for several weeks. Unfortunately, I developed a fairly deep burn during this period when I was unable to have TT. Upon her return, the skin was reddish purple, the area of skin had begun to crack and peel, and all of the tissue was quite painful. Then we had a lengthy session, which was quite an intense experience. Afterward, I felt so relaxed and somewhat tingly all over. The treatment area had a cooler sensation almost immediately.

"When I got home, the skin color had not changed much and still looked like a deep burn. I went to bed disappointed that I didn't receive the miraculous healing that I'd experienced the first time. Yet the next day, I began to experience sharp multidirectional pains throughout the treatment area. It was very intense, as if something was trying to escape from my body. In two days, the skin had a significant color change. The amount of redness was greatly reduced, except in one or two spots where it was quite red with a grayish tone. The majority of the area looked like a bruise that was well into healing, and that healing continued rapidly for several days.

"I was thrilled by these results and called the therapist for additional TT sessions to help accelerate the process. Three weeks after stopping radiation, the burn was essentially healed. While this is a shorter time frame then the doctor had suggested, I feel the progress was greatly enhanced using TT.

"Following radiation, the doctor said that I would have a skin-color change, something like a strange-looking tan that could linger for up to two years. In my case, I could clearly see the outline of the radiation area during the period of the burn. Following multiple TT sessions, the skin color became more and more normal-looking. After having a total of ten TT sessions, the skin color was essentially normal."

REIKI: THE UNIVERSAL LIFE FORCE ENERGY

What Is It?

Reiki, the Japanese word for universal life-force energy, is a technique for stress reduction and relaxation that allows everyone to tap into an unlimited supply of life-force energy to improve health and enhance the quality of life.

Where Did It Come From?

Rei means universal, and *ki* means the same as Qi in Chinese, prana in Sanskrit, and *ti* or *ki* in Hawaiian. This energy-based touch therapy was practiced thousands of years ago in the Buddhist monasteries of Tibet. In the late 1880s, it was rediscovered by a Christian minister, Dr. Mikao Usul, who was interested in the ancient healing arts; it was brought to this country by Hawayo Takata in the 1940s.

How Does It Work?

With Reiki, energy enters the practitioner through the top of the head and exits through the hands, being directed into the body or energy field of the recipient. Reiki is a very subtle form of healing and may be done through clothing and without any physical contact between the practitioner and client. The practitioner places her or his hands on or near the client's body in a series of positions. Each position, whether on the hands, feet, or shoulders, is held for three to ten minutes, depending on how much Reiki the client needs. The entire treatment usually lasts between forty to ninety minutes.

What's It Good For?

If used effectively, Reiki can boost energy, healing, and mental clarity and decrease pain. It is used to heal headaches, stomachaches, bee stings, colds, flu, tension, and anxiety; it also helps reduce the side effects of medical treatments for serious illness, including chemotherapy. Most patients experience stress reduction with some improvement in physical and psychological condition.

Where's the Science?

An intriguing study in the journal *Cancer Prevention and Control* (1997) gives an example of how Reiki can be used effectively for health and healing. Researchers set out to explore the usefulness of Reiki for pain relief as opposed to narcotic medications. Twenty volunteers participated in the study and were treated by a second-degree Reiki practitioner. Pain was monitored before and after the Reiki treatment using a visual analogue scale and a Likert scale. Using these measurements, researchers found that there was a great reduction in pain following the Reiki treatment.

Credentials

As with other types of touch therapies, proper training is necessary for practicing Reiki. The practitioner training is usually taught in three levels, with a series of teachings at each level. These levels are taught in workshops followed by hands-on practice. After completing each level of training, students receive certification.

Astonishing Healing Is Documented
"The Lump Had Shrunk by a Centimeter, Was Soft, Freely Mobile, and Not Tender."

Dr. Daniel J. Benor, a holistic psychiatrist in Philadelphia, tells of accepting an invitation to observe Ethel Lombardi, a Reiki healing master. "This challenge changed my life. Ethel brought about a physical change in a young man that was impossible, according to all my medical and psychological understanding of how the body functions. A lump under his nipple started out measuring one by two centimeters, was rubbery-firm [like an eraser], was more mixed than one would like to see in any lump [suggesting it might be invasive], and was quite tender. Ethel treated him with a laying on of hands, placing her hands over the chakras—the energy centers on the midline of the body. After only half an hour, during which time the young man cried vigorously, without explaining what he was experiencing [that bothered me, as a psychiatrist!], the lesion had changed. It had shrunk by a centimeter, was soft, freely mobile, and not tender.

"Fortunately, another physician was there with me, and we agreed on our palpation of the lesion before and after the healing. Otherwise, I am certain I would have let what we call retrocognitive dissonance convince me that I must have mismeasured or misremembered my perceptions—in order to explain away something that contradicted my expectations and understandings of what can happen with a lump under a young man's nipple in half an hour."

UNRAVELING THE MYSTERY OF
ENERGY-BASED THERAPIES

While it's difficult to understand energy-based therapies, the fact that they frequently lead to healing astounds many. But just as science could not understand early on how a potent pharmaceutical could treat cardiovascular disease or cancer, researchers are only beginning to comprehend the perplexing mysteries of energy-based healing. Give science a few more years, and the chances are great that therapeutic touch and Reiki will become widely recommended to reduce the deleterious effects of stress.

CHAPTER SEVEN

Aromas, Oils, and Essences: Natural Ways to Boost Healing

IF THE DAY AND NIGHT ARE SUCH THAT YOU GREET THEM WITH JOY AND
LIFE EMITS A FRAGRANCE LIKE FLOWERS AND SWEET SCENTED HERBS—
THAT IS YOUR SUCCESS. ALL NATURE IS YOUR CONGRATULATIONS.
—*Henry David Thoreau*

When Mary Alice Postula, a registered nurse at a private nursing home in California, began giving aromatherapy massages to ten men and women with Alzheimer's disease, she had no idea what the results would be. Yet after rubbing their delicate skin with essence of jasmine and lemon for thirty minutes, three times a week for six weeks, the patients were more responsive, and four even acknowledged family members again.

Why is the power of smell such a forceful trigger to the human nervous system? There is no denying that certain aromas, such as homemade chocolate chip cookies, a freshly brewed cappuccino, or freshly cut grass, can elicit comforting memories of days gone by. For some people, simply hearing the words "fudge" or "gingerbread" can cause them to salivate in anticipation of the real thing. This is because different aromas have such arousing smells that when they reach the brain via the nose, the brain reacts with a dramatic change of mood, emotion, or even overall alertness.

Different aromas, essences, or oils are said to have specific healing powers: They can reduce anxiety, combat stress, fight infection, increase productivity, or serve as powerful aphrodisiacs. For example, lavender and spiced apples are said to increase the alpha-wave activity in the back of the brain, which leads to relaxation and feelings of contentment. Increased beta activity in the front of the brain shows greater alertness and is said to occur with the scents of lemon or jasmine. Because most aromas have an immediate effect, certain odors, such as smelling salts, can instantly revive someone who is feeling faint.

Therapeutic massage with aromatherapy oils heightens the healing effect. There are a host of natural aromas, oils, and essences that are used with touch or energy-based therapies to reduce stress, anxiety, and insomnia, in addition to supporting healing. For example, with bodywork or massage, friction on the skin is reduced by using oil, powders, or even cornstarch.

AROMATHERAPY

What Is It?
Aromatherapy is complementary healing that uses fragrances or essential and absolute oils and other substances for physical and psychological benefits. While aromatherapy is commonly used for pleasure, such as with scented candles, baths, or fragrances, it is also used for medicinal purposes. Massage therapists, nurses, and some conventional medical doctors use aromatherapy in conjunction with other treatment modalities. Dawn Bennett, M.D., a family practitioner in Ohio, uses peppermint and eucalyptus oil to alleviate chest tightness and reduce mucus production in adults with respiratory problems.

Essential Oils Are Highly Concentrated and Aromatic
Essential oils are highly concentrated substances extracted from different parts of a plant, including the flower, bark, roots, leaves, wood, resin, seeds, or rind (in the case of citrus fruits). The oils

contain healing vitamins, antibiotics, and antiseptics and represent the life force of the plant.

Scientists agree that essential oils may perform more than one function in living plants. In some cases they seem to be a part of the plant's immune system. In other cases they may simply be end products of metabolism. Essential oils contain hundreds of organic constituents, including hormones, vitamins, and other natural elements that work on many levels. For example, essential oils can be sedative or stimulating. Some are antispasmodic, and most are antibacterial. Essential oils are seventy-five to a hundred times more concentrated than the oils in dried herbs.

Carrier Oils Provide Lubrication

Carrier oils are used to make essential oils suitable for massage. Essential oils are too powerful to be used undiluted on the skin. Carrier oils provide good lubrication for a massage therapist's hands to glide over a patient's skin surface. They are health-giving substances in their own right, carrying healing vitamins, and minerals. They support the skin's ability to function, to breathe, and to absorb light. Carrier oils also help to regulate the skin's temperature, soften the skin, and give the skin elasticity. Rubbing aromatic oil into the skin can be either calming or stimulating, depending on the type of oil used.

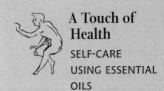

A Touch of Health

SELF-CARE USING ESSENTIAL OILS

- Inhale the oil by adding five to ten drops to steaming water or to a humidifier.
- Mix one teaspoon oil with one pint carrier oil, and use as a massage oil.
- Add five to ten drops to warm bathwater.
- Mix five drops with one cup warm water and mist into the air.
- Put one to two drops on top of a candle's melted wax, and inhale the warm scent.

Commonly Used Carrier Oils

Aloe vera	Olive oil
Apricot	Passionflower
Avocado	Peachnut
Borage	Rapeseed
Calendula	Rose hip
Camellia	Safflower
Carrot seed	Sesame seed
Evening primrose	Soy
Grape seed	St.-John's-wort
Hazelnut	Sunflower
Jojoba	Sweet almond
Kernel	Walnut
Macadamia	Wheat germ
Mineral oil	

Where Did It Come From?

Since the beginning of civilization, combinations of oils, fragrant plants, and resins were used in some form, whether for medicinal or ceremonial purposes. Early traders carried plants and aromatic oils along the established routes of ancient civilizations. Aromatherapy was used in Egypt more than three thousand years ago to cure illness. Ancient Egyptians also used aromatic plants and oils for massage, embalming, and cosmetics. During the reign of the Egyptian pharaoh Khufu, papyrus manuscripts recorded the use of fragrant herbs, perfumes, and temple incense, and told of healing salves made of fragrant resins. The most famous Egyptian fragrance, *kyphi* (or "welcome to the gods"), was said to induce hypnotic states.

There are biblical records of herbal use in the Middle East

from over two thousand years ago, particularly the fragrant herbs myrrh and frankincense. Accounts tell of the ancient Hebrews using aromatherapy fragrances to consecrate their temples, altars, and priests. In fact, the Bible's Book of Exodus in the Old Testament gives the recipe for the holy anointing oil given to Moses to initiate priests: a blend of myrrh, cinnamon, and calamus, mixed with olive oil.

Aromatherapy was commonly used in Greece. Before going to battle, Greek warriors anointed themselves with oils, and by the seventh century B.C., hundreds of perfumers set up shops in the mercantile center of Athens. Aromatherapy was used in early Rome, where clients would be massaged with oil after taking a bath.

During the Middle Ages in Europe, such plants as cypress, clove, and rosemary were burned to help control the plague. The use of aromatherapy moved to the Far East, and upper classes in China made lavish use of fragrance. Not only did they use fragrances on their bodies and clothing, but their homes and temples were all richly scented, as were ink, paper, and tiny sachets tucked into their garments. Some of the most commonly used aromas were jasmine—which was used as a general tonic—rose, to improve digestion; chamomile to reduce headaches and colds; and ginger to fight coughs and treat malaria.

Even though incense didn't arrive in Japan until around 500 A.D., the Japanese turned the use of incense into a fine art, having perfected a distillation process. Incense was burned for ceremonial purposes, and students performed story dances for incense-burning rituals.

On the other side of the world, the Aztecs used aromas and essence for medicinal purposes, massaging injured warriors with scented salves in the sweat lodges. Massage ointments of valerian and other herbs were made by the Incas, and the Mayans in Central America steamed their patients in cramped clay structures.

Native Americans used aromatherapy in more traditional

ways, using steam to treat congestion, chronic pain, headaches, fainting, and other problems. Echinacea, an herb commonly used today, was used as a smoke treatment for migraines or headaches.

Even though this complement to touch therapy has strong ancient roots, it was not actually given a name until the 1930s. The term "aromatherapy" comes from the French word *aroma-thérapie*, coined by René-Maurice Gattefossé, a chemist whose book of the same name was published in 1928. After a lab explosion, Gattefossé conveniently plunged his injured hand into a container of lavender oil and was amazed by how quickly it healed. Two French homeopaths, Dr. Jean Valnet and the Austrian-born biochemist Marguerite Maury, were inspired by Gattefossé's work. In the 1960s, Valnet, an army surgeon, used essential oils such as thyme, clove, lemon, and chamomile on wounds and burns, and he later found fragrances successful in treating psychiatric problems.

How Does It Work?

Smell has been a primary determinant of basic behavior since the beginning of the evolutionary cycle, yet the workings of aromatherapy still remain a mystery to even the most astute of scientists. Researchers do know that aromatic molecules are received by the cilia, or fine hairs, linked to the olfactory nerve and then to the brain. Olfactory cells are found in a tiny piece of tissue high up in your nose. They connect directly to your brain and let you distinguish the fragrance of homemade bread, baby powder, and fresh-brewed coffee—that is, when you can breathe through your nose. This message is received in the limbic system, the oldest or most primitive part of the brain, which has been called the emotional switchboard of the brain. Your emotions and memory are processed in the limbic system of the brain, and stimulation of this system is considered a direct pathway to influencing your mood, emotions, and overall alertness. Because the limbic system is directly connected to the parts of the brain that control heart rate, blood pressure, breathing, memory, stress levels, and hormone balance, scientists have learned that oil fragrances may be one of the fastest ways to bring about physiological or psychological effects. Either stimulation or sedation of body systems or organs may occur.

Some believe that the oils, when used in a bath or massage, are absorbed through the skin and carried by body fluids to the main body systems—such as the nervous and muscular systems—for a healing effect.

What Are the Different Types of Aromatherapy?
The different types of aromatherapy are cosmetic, massage, and olfactory. Regardless of which type of aromatherapy you choose, essential oils should always be diluted in a carrier oil or water.

- *Cosmetic aromatherapy* combines essential oils with facial, skin, body, and hair-care products.

- *Massage aromatherapy* combines the healing touch of massage therapy with the aromatic benefits of essential oils.

- *Olfactory aromatherapy* releases essential oils into the environment around you either by inhaling or diffusion. For inhalation, you can either dispense the essential oil into a handkerchief or spray a mixture of essential oils and distilled water into the air and breathe in. Diffusion is the evaporation of the aromatic components of an oil into the atmosphere using aromatherapy equipment.

What's It Good For?
The alleged benefits of aromatherapy range from stress relief to enhancement of immunity and the unlocking of emotions from

past experiences. Many oils have proven antiseptic properties and can be used as first aid and as an ongoing treatment for cuts, burns, insect bites, and bruises. Some other oils are anti-inflammatory, antibacterial, and antibiotic, among many other properties. Oils with antifungal properties can be used to treat fungal infections such as athlete's foot. Some can aid in the overall management of more serious conditions, such as candida (yeast infection), arthritis, and chronic pain.

Where's the Science?

A recent report in *The Lancet*, a well-respected medical journal, indicated that lavender oil could possibly replace hypnotic drugs used for insomnia in the elderly. Some of these drugs could have side effects and have been prescribed for ongoing periods of time. Although the number of people in the study was small, geriatric residents of a nursing home who had been prescribed tranquilizers for a couple of years had their sleep measured for six weeks. The medication was used the first two weeks and discontinued the next two; the ward was perfumed with a diffuser and lavender oil the last two weeks. It seemed that although removing the medication reduced the number of hours spent sleeping, the scent of lavender restored the time to that obtained through medication. Residents also appeared less restless during sleep.

A study reported in the *Indian Journal of Medical Research* (December 2000) found that oil massage, particularly sesame oil, improved infants' growth and helped them sleep better. Oil massage is a time-tested method of infant care practiced all over the world and is known to have beneficial effects. In this study, researchers from the University College of Medical Sciences in Delhi studied the effect of oil massage on 125 healthy infants. The infants were approximately six weeks of age and were divided into five groups. Four groups received oil massage with herbal oil, sesame oil, mustard oil, and a mix of mineral oil with vitamin E, respectively. The fifth group served as the control and did not receive any massage.

In the study, the mothers were taught to massage the infants' legs, back, arms, chest, abdomen, face, and head with oil for a total of ten minutes daily. This practice was continued over a period of four weeks. After the study, researchers noted that the weight, body length, head circumference, and girth of arms and legs were increased in the four groups that received oil massage, and the most significant increase was seen in the group that received massage with sesame oil. A significant increase in the blood flow through the femoral artery, the main artery supplying the leg, was also seen in this group. Researchers found the infants who received the oil massage also slept better. The beneficial effects on growth and sleep are probably due to increased blood flow and increase in levels of growth promoting hormones like growth hormone and insulin.

Other studies confirm aromatherapy's special power to change mood or emotion:

- In a study published in the *International Journal of Neuroscience* (Volume 96, 1998), adults exposed to rosemary showed decreased alpha and beta brain waves, suggesting increased alertness. They also had lower anxiety levels and performed math computations faster. Adults exposed to lavender showed increased beta power, suggesting increased relaxation. They performed math computations not only faster but also with fewer errors.

- A study in *Headache Quarterly* (Volume 9, 1998) reported on the effects of inhaling green-apple fragrance to reduce the severity of migraine headaches. The researchers theorized that since certain ambient odors reduce anxiety, green-apple aroma may affect emotions positively in other contexts, helping to reduce the severity of migraine symptoms during an attack. Fifty patients were asked to rate the severity of their headaches at the onset and ten minutes later during three separate headache episodes. The first and third episodes served as controls, but during the second headache episode, the subjects sniffed green-apple fragrance from an inhaler. The resulting data indicated that green-apple aroma may be useful as an auxiliary therapy in managing chronic headache.

* In a study done in London, England, researchers studied the effects on brain-wave patterns when essential oils are inhaled or smelled. They found that oils such as orange, jasmine, and rose have a tranquilizing effect by altering the brain waves into a rhythm that produces calmness. Furthermore, stimulating oils—basil, black pepper, rosemary, and cardamom—work by producing a heightened energy response.

* A study in the *Pre and Perinatal Psychology Journal* reported that infants showed fewer stress behaviors (grimacing and clenched fists) after being massaged with oil, as opposed to a dry massage.

Using Aromatherapy with Massage

Massage encourages relaxation as well as circulation, and eases minor aches and pains. Some believe that when aromatherapy is combined with massage, essential oils are absorbed and used by the skin and body. You can use the following oils as inhalation, or with massage, self-massage, or in a soothing aromatherapy bath.

* *Lavender:* Heals burns and cuts; destroys bacteria; relieves inflammation, spasms, headaches, respiratory allergies, muscle aches, nausea, menstrual cramps
* *Peppermint:* Alleviates digestive problems; cleans wounds; decongests the chest; relieves headache, neuralgia, and muscle pain

- *Eucalyptus*: Clears sinuses; has antibacterial and antiviral properties; relieves coughs
- *Rosemary*: Relieves pain; increases circulation; decongests the chest; reduces swelling
- *Chamomile*: Reduces swelling; treats allergic symptoms; relieves stress, insomnia, and depression; useful in treating digestive problems
- *Thyme*: Lessens laryngitis and coughs; fights skin infections; relieves pain in the joints
- *Tarragon*: Stimulates digestion; calms neural and digestive tracts; relieves menstrual symptoms and stress
- *Everlasting*: Heals scars; reduces swelling after injuries; relieves sunburn; treats pain from arthritis, muscle injuries, sprains and strains, tendinitis

FLOWER ESSENCE THERAPY

What Is It?

Flower essences are liquid plant extracts charged with the electromagnetic pattern of specific flowers; they are used by natural therapists to restore mental, emotional, and spiritual well-being.

Where Did It Come From?

Edward Bach (1886–1936), a medical doctor, bacteriologist, and homeopathic physician, dedicated his life to discovering a system of healing that would go beyond the diagnosis and treatment of physical symptoms to the emotional and mental roots of disease. Bach realized that when people were treated on the basis of distinctive personality characteristics, rather than according to their disease, true healing could occur. Convinced that he would find what he sought in nature, he began to explore the fields and forests of England in search of remedies that would be effective, pure, and inexpensive.

Bach theorized that the heat of the sun, acting through the dew, must draw out the healing essence of each flower. He then developed a way to extract this essence and experimented to isolate flowers that addressed a range of psychological conditions; thus the Bach Flower Remedies. Each of the thirty-eight remedies strengthens the person to dissolve the energy blockages, a similar philosophy to other holistic therapies.

How Does It Work?

Essences of flowers are diluted and preserved in brandy and then diluted with water. Usually the dose of a Bach Flower Remedy is a few drops taken either sublingually (under the tongue) or mixed with a few ounces of water and swallowed. Sometimes essences are rubbed into the skin during a massage or used on the practitioner's hands during an energy-based healing treatment, such as Reiki.

While pharmaceutical drugs mask or alleviate negative physical symptoms, Bach flower essences address the emotional imbalances that create disease. They operate on the principle that if a person has a problem, she or he has, deep within, the virtue to counteract it. For example, if you lack confidence, you have a blockage that prevents the natural feelings of high self-esteem from surfacing. In taking the essence, you are overwhelmed with feelings of confidence, and the blockage that was hindering you is gone.

What's It Good For?

Dr. Bach wanted his remedies to be simple so anyone could use these without consulting a healthcare professional. Some popular remedies include agrimony to treat hidden mental torture and elm for feelings of being overwhelmed. There is also a combination remedy called Rescue Remedy, a blend of Cherry Plum, Clematis, Impatiens, Rock Rose, and Star of Bethlehem, that treats multiple stress disorders.

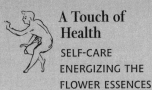

A Touch of Health

SELF-CARE
ENERGIZING THE
FLOWER ESSENCES

Flower Essences and Reiki

Master teacher Cheryl Strope tells of using flower essences in her Reiki practice: "Over the course of my usage with this blend of healing therapies, there have consistently been before-and-after distinctions in the session experience. Some are very subtle and detectable by clients, while others are only momentarily detectable by the changes in the Reiki stream flowing through my hands. I treated a seventeen-year-old who was playing high school football. Three days before the playoffs, he injured his ankle during practice. Hoping he would be able to play in the game that Friday, his mother, a Reiki student, made an appointment for him to see me. When he arrived, I asked him to remove his shoe and sock, something unusual for Reiki work, so I could directly apply drops of Star of Bethlehem (for trauma), Five-Flower Formula (to ensure vitality in the area), and Self-heal (to accelerate healing). Along with direct topical application, I also put drops of those flower essences into my palms. I applied three special Reiki techniques along with additional Reiki on the injured ankle. Before

When you use flower essences purchased at natural-food stores, be sure to energize the bottled essence for full effectiveness. Cheryl Stroup, a California-based Reiki master teacher, says, "All applications of flower essences call for potentizing before use and are done with the essence at the stock level. By lightly tapping or shaking the bottle before using it, you can ensure that the matrix pattern is energized at the time of dispensing. Flower essences may receive Reiki attunements in their original packaging with an effect similar to attuning anything else. The attuned flower essence would then channel the Reiki stream in the bottle, as well as all particles dispersed in any of the usage formats.

"A Reiki master will simply hold the bottle between her hands and run the Reiki stream as a thank-you to the flowers, as well as to enhance the life force within the imprint pattern of the essence. Simply put, this means that all levels of effectiveness and traits contained within the flower essence are animated with vital force as an autonomous life form."

leaving, I gave him some Star of Bethlehem and suggested he apply the remedy to his ankle four times a day, especially after getting out of any water. I also suggested an additional Reiki session in two days.

"Upon arising the next morning, he said, much of the swelling was gone. Although there was some pain, he could walk without a cane. At school that afternoon, he soaked his ankle in a whirlpool. When he came to see me on Thursday evening, I repeated the same procedures as the prior session and sent him on his way. On Friday, he was walking pain-free, and with his ankle taped, he was able to play in the entire game. His team won, to everyone's delight!

"Whether or not such results can be pinned down in a linear format, however, is questionable, since awareness is also governed by an individual's sensitivity to energy. Nonetheless, I continue to use flower essences when so compelled.

"For a regular session with a client, I usually put two to four drops of an essence on my hands and rub them together to distribute the flower essence pattern. This also decreases the liquid form at the same time. The pattern of the flower essences is retained on the hands for a period of time. The Reiki stream emphasizes whatever attributes and correlated healing specialties are pertinent to the client, in priority item order, while orchestrating the process for maximum impact. How long one can distinctly perceive a flower essence's influence varies, and there is no consistency from one case to another. However, because the flower essence patterns seem to work in a similar fashion as the Reiki keys, i.e., their characteristics coincide with a particular harmonic resonance chord pattern within the Reiki stream itself, I simply allow the wisdom of the Reiki source to determine the flower essence's patterned activity period. To this date, there have been no ill effects reported to me.

"Because the process by which flower essences work is governed largely by mutual resonance, there are really no side or ill effects from their use, even if a given essence currently has no therapeutic value for this particular soul. I generally inform clients when I would like to apply a flower essence to my hands during the session, and tell them what the potential benefits are. For example, Self-heal flower essence helps orchestrate and enhance the client's individual healing capabilities on all levels. When Self-heal essence is used with the Reiki stream, quality, activation, and integration of these individual healing characteristics seem to be more easily available. Because of the brandy preservative, I will usually apply the essences after I do the hands-over-the-eyes position. This way, the leftover alcohol scent is not directly inhaled by the client.

"For a client with a physical ailment, depending on the anatomical area of complaint, I may topically apply the flower essences as I did in the sprained-ankle case I mentioned earlier. If the location is more intimate, I will simply place the drops in my palms and apply them about one to one and a half inches above the physical body while the drops are still wet. For other situations, I will place the drops in my palms and invoke keys using the physical-drawing option while the essence is still damp. Because of the energy-field construct, this delivery method will also have a definite impact.

"I treated a fifty-year-old woman with severe shoulder, arm, and elbow pain. Arm movement was severely limited much of the time. Conventional medical treatment was not providing her with any substantial or long-term relief. She had previously taken Reiki classes with me, and since she had experienced total pain relief from her class sessions, she decided to try Reiki again. During the first session, I applied blackberry flower essence to my hands as I worked at her shoulder area. Blackberry helps move energy into the limbs. At our second session, I was intuitively aware of heart injuries contributing to the distress and pain, so I applied nicotiana (for numbed emotions and sensitivity) and pine (for guilt) to my hands while running Reiki on the upper body, both front and back. At the conclusion of this session, her pain rating went from a five to zero. She still has good days and bad days, though she no longer has any pain in her elbow, arm, or wrist. We continue to work with the shoulder area as her schedule permits."

Using Flower Essences Topically

Paul Wyman is a certified massage-therapy teacher who has been in private practice for eight years. As a proponent of using flower essences topically, Wyman has achieved "impressive healing results" in the reduction of scar tissue pain, temporomandibular joint syndrome (TMJ), and arthritis. He believes undiluted drops directly from the stock bottle work the best, and he chooses essences by muscle testing. "I used Star of Bethlehem on an enormous scar on the torso of a Vietnam veteran. By applying the drops topically, the scar tissue went from being tight, white, painful, and restrictive of motion to a full range of motion with no pain. The scar itself was reduced to about half its previous size. I did not use massage or any other therapy. I can't prove it, but I believe the essence dissolved the scar tissue. It was absolutely astonishing. I kept a photographic record of the case."

Wyman cites cases of clients with bursitis and arthritis who, after receiving a few drops of holly, zinnia, and/or spinach essences discovered their joints had loosened up and much of the pain had gone. Wyman also uses the Self-heal cream with these clients. "The arthritis clients I work on find it extremely helpful. I have them put a few drops of an essence in the cream and rub it into the joints. Any time there is a need for skin involvement with an energy disturbance, I always use Self-heal cream."

He notes that clients who are taking antidepressant drugs do not seem to receive the positive effects of flower essences. "I have a few patients who are on fairly high doses of antidepressants and have been unable to perceive much effect from essences. I think the drugs have a blanketing effect which profoundly blocks the energy movements."

The first flower essence Wyman used topically was agrimony, for chronic TMJ. He put a few drops on the affected area, and the next day the client threw away the bite guard she had been using for twenty years. "It made sense her TMJ would be helped by agrimony because of the profile of the essence; someone who is always smiling, trying to show a cheerful side of themselves, but not willing to show any other feelings. If one is smiling all the time, the jaw would be the place where tension would manifest itself."

Wyman often sends clients home with an essence to continue the treatment orally. He calls Star of Bethlehem "an astonishing remedy for topical application, because it releases cellular memory. Much of what happens occurs physically and then is kept in the memory. We hold so much shock in our bodies from experiences, and it can get trapped there. At times it seems all roads lead to Star of Bethlehem."

A HEALING COMBINATION

Combining any touch therapy with aromatic essences and oils serves to boost optimal health. Find the fragrances that work best for you, whether they are oil of essences massaged gently into your skin or Bach flower remedies carefully chosen to help you resolve personal emotional issues. After all, who's to say that these alternative therapies are not part of our intended "natural" cure? Aromas, oils, and essences are the precious gifts of nature that we can access any time to use for healing and wholeness.

CHAPTER EIGHT

Imagine Yourself Well

GREAT MEN ARE THEY WHO SEE THAT SPIRITUAL IS STRONGER THAN ANY
MATERIAL FORCE, THAT THOUGHTS RULE THE WORLD.

—*Ralph Waldo Emerson*

Ask any qualified touch therapists how to achieve optimal health, and most will say, "Take personal responsibility for yourself." Now, this doesn't mean memorizing your doctor's phone number so you can quickly get the latest pharmaceutical "cure." Rather, it means making responsible and healthy lifestyle choices every day—carefully selecting what you eat, what you do, the friends you spend time with, the amount of exercise and sleep you get, and what you think.

"Can what you think really affect personal health?" you might ask. Absolutely! A new school of medicine called psychoneuroimmunology (PNI), or the study of how the mind and body interplay, is based on the premise that mental or emotional processes affect physiologic function. Health professionals in this field figure that between 90 and 95 percent of all health problems can be traced to the influence of emotions. Some are going so far as to say that an optimistic outlook, such as a feeling of control, may in some way protect against disease or illness and act as a valuable complement to conventional medical care. While alternative medicine has no scientific validation, mind/body interventions are scientifically proven, with a foundation in traditional medicine such as surgery and pharmaceuticals.

Those on the cutting edge of PNI contend that many influences are at work in each of us to either keep us well or allow us to get sick. Scientific evidence suggests that such factors as stress, negative feelings, and lack of social support can influence immune status and function, as well as speed disease onset and progression. Although still early in its development, research suggests psychological factors may play a role in autoimmune diseases like allergies, arthritis, and multiple sclerosis.

In the 1970s, Harvard cardiologist Herbert Benson, M.D., author of *The Relaxation Response* and founder of the Mind Body Medical Institute, was the first physician to scientifically document the physiological benefits of meditation through his studies with experienced transcendental meditators. As one of the great pioneers of mind/body medicine, Benson helped to explain PNI, suggesting that the practice of medicine is like a three-legged stool, where the legs of surgery and medications are balanced with spiritual self-care. This means that while medical science is crucial for keeping us well, the mind/body connection may be equally important in staving off illness altogether.

Thanks to the early theories of Benson and other brilliant researchers, many studies are now focused on the connections between these areas, particularly the mechanisms by which the mind and emotions affect physical well-being. For someone who can't shake a lingering cold, or is concerned about an increased risk for heart disease, cancer, or diabetes, these lifesaving studies can outline how emotional distress may be a crucial barrier to wellness.

THE PITFALLS OF STRESS

As explained in Chapter 1, stress activates the sympathetic nervous system, stimulating the release of hormones such as cortisol. A constant saturation of these hormones results in many physiologic changes, including increased heart rate, breathing, and blood pressure. Under normal conditions, these changes subside quickly, but chronic stressors—including anxiety, fear, anger, and grief—can keep the nervous system perpetually aroused. Prolonged stress has been found to contribute to illness and immune changes in both human and animal models.

Given the evidence that stress contributes to illness, it seems logical to presume that decreasing stress can modulate illness. The most convincing evidence appears in *Archives of General Psychiatry*, which cites two small but well-done studies by researchers at the UCLA School of Medicine. One six-month study found that malignant melanoma patients trained in relaxation techniques showed significant increases in the number and activity of cancer-slaying natural killer cells; the recently published six-year follow-up found higher mortality among the untrained group. This is where bodywork and energy-based therapies can help. Most touch therapies are based on the premise that the mind and body are interconnected to an extent far surpassing previous assumptions, and that physical health and emotional well-being are closely linked. Touch therapies can increase endorphins and enable you to experience positive feelings; reports suggest that using mind/body exercises along with various types of bodywork can boost these feelings and that these benefits extend throughout the entire day.

We all know that when we have peaceful thoughts, we tend to have a comparable emotional reaction and similar physiological reaction; we feel in control of our life and our health. When we have angry or anxious thoughts, we tend to be emotionally aroused, and our physiological reactions are consequently more dramatic, which makes us prone to bad health choices. An increasing number of physicians, psychiatrists, and psychologists are acknowledging that the way we think, feel, act, and react can be a powerful determinant of physical and mental health.

Understanding the Relaxation Response

In his studies, Dr. Herbert Benson found that there was a counterbalancing mechanism to the fight-or-flight response. Just stimulating an area of the hypothalamus can cause the stress response, but activating other areas of the brain results in its reduction. This study led to the discovery of the relaxation response, a physiological state of inner quiet and peacefulness, a calming of negative thoughts and worries, and a mental focus away from the pain itself. There are many techniques to elicit the relaxation response, which are explained later on.

Relaxation is defined by decreased muscle tension and respiration, lower blood pressure and heart rate, and improved circulation. The relaxation response slows down the sympathetic nervous system, leading to:

+ Decreased heart rate
+ Decreased blood pressure
+ Decreased sweat production
+ Decreased oxygen consumption
+ Decreased catecholamine production (dopamine and norepinephrine, or brain chemicals associated with the stress response)
+ Decreased cortisol (stress hormone) production

Eliciting the relaxation response in conjunction with massage or other touch therapies is an added bonus in reducing emotional stress of daily living. Once you've learned the physiological process of relaxing, you can summon this decrease in sympathetic arousal with many different interventions, such as progressive muscle relaxation, meditation, guided imagery, and music therapy.

Some people experience benefits from mind/body tools within minutes of doing them. For example, deep abdominal breathing actually alters your psychological state, diminishing the intensity

A Touch of Health

START WITH FIFTEEN MINUTES A DAY

To begin your own relaxation program, set aside a period of about fifteen minutes that you can devote solely to relaxation practice. Choose a time when you have few obligations or commitments, so you won't feel hurried or rushed. Remove outside distractions that can disrupt your concentration: Turn off the radio, the television, even the ringer on the telephone.

During practice, it is important to either lie flat or recline comfortably so that your whole body is supported, relieving as much tension or tightness in your muscles as you can. During the fifteen minutes remain as still as possible; try to direct your thoughts away from the events of the day, focusing on the immediate moment. Observe only yourself and the different feelings or sensations you may notice throughout your body. Can you tell which parts of your body feel relaxed and loose, and which parts feel tense and uptight?

There are two essential steps to eliciting the relaxation response:

1. Repetition of a word, sound, phrase, prayer, or muscular activity
2. Passive disregard of everyday thoughts that inevitably come to mind and the return to your repetition

PICTURE YOUR BODY AT PEACE

As you go through the relaxation steps, try to visualize every muscle in your body becoming loose, relaxed, and free of any excess tension. Picture your muscles beginning to unwind; imagine them going loose and limp. As you do this, breathe evenly and slowly, as if with each breath you melt the tension away.

At the end of the session, examine your feelings and sensations. Notice whether areas that felt tight at first now feel more loose and relaxed, and whether any areas of tension remain. Don't be surprised if the relaxed feeling begins to dissipate once you return to normal activities. It's usually only after several weeks of daily, consistent practice that you can maintain the relaxed feeling beyond the practice session itself.

of a stressful moment. Think about how your respiration quickens when you are fearful. Then consider how taking a deep, slow breath brings an immediate calming effect. Likewise, music therapy can lessen your heart rate on the first experience, if you mindfully focus on the music, rhythm, and resulting inner peace.

Learning to Relax

Relaxation can offer a real potential to reduce physical strain and emotional, negative thoughts—and increase your ability to self-manage stress. Achieving relaxation uses a mental approach to activity in general rather than any one specific activity. For each of us, many different activities or routines may be relaxing, depending on our particular mind-set, and what may be relaxing for one person can be frustrating or tension-producing for another. For example, some of us may find it calming and soothing to lie quietly and listen to a certain type of music; others may gain more relaxation from reading an enjoyable book.

Combination Therapy Helps to Reduce Pain

In a study at the University of Florida, researchers concluded that massage may help patients with sickle cell anemia, an inherited disorder of hemoglobin, the oxygen-carrying molecule in red blood cells. Results from their pilot study comparing massage and relaxation therapy show that both techniques safely and effectively reduced pain.

Because relaxation is a physiological reaction that causes blood vessels to dilate, improving blood flow, researchers believe this might keep sickle cells from blocking vessels. Also, massage may move blood through vessels via stroking. In the study, sixteen people with sickle cell anemia were assigned either six thirty-minute massage sessions or to learn relaxation techniques at weekly meetings that would help them cope with their pain. At the end of each session, patients also engaged in a five-minute visualization exercise that focused on relaxation.

Researchers recorded pain levels and participants' ability to function before and after the study, and both massage and relaxation appeared to help. The sixteen participants reported significant reductions in the amount of pain they experienced even after just one session. In some cases, the massage or relaxation response cut their pain intensity in half.

Researchers believe that massage might increase the body's natural production of the brain chemical serotonin, which is associated with pain relief.

After you learn the relaxation response, incorporate this state of mind in the following mind/body techniques. Each can be used in conjunction with touch therapies—either before, during, or after massage, bodywork, or energy-based healing.

PROGRESSIVE MUSCLE RELAXATION

What Is It?

Progressive muscle relaxation involves concentrating on different muscle groups as you relax. This mindfulness, or focus of attention on what you feel from moment to moment, can help you move beyond destructive habits as you become centered in a world of health and inner peace.

Where Did It Come From?

Progressive muscle relaxation was developed by Dr. Edmund Jacobson more than fifty years ago. Jacobson discovered that by tensing and releasing various muscle groups throughout the body, you would go into a deep state of relaxation. While Jacobson originally developed a series of 200 different relaxation exercises, this has been shortened to fifteen to twenty exercises, which are just as effective in reducing tension and anxiety.

How Does It Work?

Lying comfortably on your back in a peaceful environment, with or without soothing music, contract then relax all of the major muscle groups in the body. Starting with your head, neck, shoulders, and arms, tense these muscles to a slow count of ten, then release them slowly to the count of ten. Now progress to your chest, back, stomach, pelvis, legs, and feet, again tensing and releasing the muscles to a slow count of ten. It is important to breathe deeply from the abdomen, focusing on your breath. Breathe in while tensing the muscles; breathe out while relaxing them.

What's It Good For?
Studies show that when you can create a strong mental image using this type of relaxation technique, you actually feel removed from cumbersome stress and negative emotions.

DEEP ABDOMINAL BREATHING

Lourdes Teaches Deep Abdominal Breathing to Aid in Relaxation
Lourdes Gonzalez believes deep abdominal breathing before massage helps to release any pent-up anxiety or tension and can help to make the massage more relaxing and healing. This thirty-one-year-old bodywork practitioner in Boca Raton, Florida, always makes sure she is centered before she begins the various strokes. She explains that "centering is a form of meditation that helps the therapist focus her energy only on that particular client.

"With massage, I focus on the *hara*, which is the center of energy in the client's abdomen. I always teach deep abdominal breathing to my client prior to the massage, so he can help me with this meditation. With soft New Age music playing in the background, my client deeply breathes in and out and becomes at peace with the world. I continue my focus and intuitively gather what problems the client is experiencing—and what challenges I have as a therapist."

Think about how your respiration quickens when you are fearful or in great pain. Taking a deep, slow breath can be calming, reducing both stress and levels of muscle pain. Breathing is one of the few activities of the body that we can consciously control, and it can measure and alter your psychological state, making a stressful moment accelerate or diminish in intensity.

What Is It?
Deep abdominal breathing is a relaxation technique that has been found to decrease the release of stress hormones and slow down your heart rate during stressful moments.

Where Did It Come From?
Deep abdominal breathing is one of the basic elements of yoga and goes back in history for thousands of years. With the thought that the breath is the bridge between the body and the mind, proper breathing (called Pranayamas) in yoga begins with taking a slow, deep breath and continuing to inhale while the abdomen and rib cage expand. You exhale in a similar way, allowing the abdomen to cave. Today deep abdominal breathing is used by many healthcare professionals and alternative medicine practitioners to help patients relax their central nervous system, slowing the heart rate, dilating the blood vessels, and causing the muscles to relax. Health gurus such as Dr. Andrew Weil, Dr. Herbert Benson, and Dr. Dean Ornish are all proponents of the healing benefit of deep breathing.

How Does It Work?
When you use deep abdominal breathing, you add oxygen to the blood and actually cause your body to release endorphins—the feel-good hormones that give a greater sense of well-being and contentment. Deep abdominal breathing can be done in conjunc-

tion with other relaxation techniques, including progressive muscle relaxation, guided imagery, and music therapy.

What's It Good For?

You can use deep abdominal breathing before and during any touch therapy, as well as times when you feel anxious or stressed. You might find it extremely helpful when you are experiencing chest tightness from anxiety. The slow deep breathing can interrupt a cycle of rapid, shallow breathing and result in less distortion of oxygen and carbon dioxide in the blood, as well as a more comfortable state of mind.

Where's the Science?

While deep abdominal breathing can be used by anyone for a calming effect, researchers are finding that it also has great benefit for those with chronic illness. In a study published in the *Journal of the American Dietetics Association* (1984), twenty-two people with cancer were assigned at random to get instruction in a certain relaxation technique, including deep abdominal breathing. Among those who completed the study, 75 percent reported a beneficial weight change over the six-week period.

Although most relaxation research has focused on pain control or stress reduction, these results suggest that relaxation may be

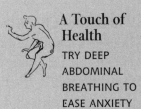

A Touch of Health

TRY DEEP ABDOMINAL BREATHING TO EASE ANXIETY

Lie comfortably on your back in a quiet room with no distractions. Place your hands on your abdomen and take in a deep, slow, deliberate breaths through your nostrils. If your hands are rising and your abdomen is expanding, then you are breathing correctly. If your hands do not rise yet your chest is rising, you are breathing incorrectly.

Inhale to a count of five, then pause for three seconds. Now exhale to a count of five. You can start with ten repetitions of this exercise; then increase to twenty-five, twice daily.

effective in treating eating problems for those with chronic illness, helping them to gain weight and increase well-being.

GUIDED IMAGERY

Jack Finally Overcomes His Fear of Flying

After a turbulent airplane ride during a horrible winter storm, forty-eight-year-old Jack Belfort of Reading, Pennsylvania, vowed never to step foot on a plane again. For most people, this pledge would not cause many problems, but it threatened Jack's livelihood. As a sales representative for a *Fortune* 500 computer-software company, he had to travel each week, from state to state in a tristate area.

For several months, Jack would leave a day early and drive to the required meetings with his company employees. This meant giving up weekends and holidays to spend time on the road—time he used to spend with his family. While this new way to commute masked Jack's fear of flying for a while, he was forced to face it again when the company CEO promoted Jack to national sales manager. The promotion meant a tremendous salary increase, but it also meant flying from coast to coast several times each month. Jack knew he'd have to overcome his fear or look for another job.

Jack sought help for this irrational fear from his internist, who recommended alternative therapies to help him learn to relax. Knowing he had to overcome this career stumbling block, Jack met with Shawn Logan, a massage therapist and counselor. As Shawn worked with Jack on learning to relax, she taught him visualization, or guided imagery. She explained to Jack how his body knew only what his mind was feeding it. Even though he was perfectly safe on the airplane, his fearful mind caused him to feel panic, increasing his heart rate and making him want to run and get off the plane.

Shawn taught Jack a way to clear his mind of unnecessary fear and clutter by immediately substituting pleasant thoughts when the fears overcame him. If he felt air turbulence while on the plane, Jack was to replace that fear with memories of sitting on the dock at his lakeside home, watching the sunset with his wife and children. Jack would visualize feeling the warm summer breeze, smelling the freshly mowed grass, tasting the iced lemonade, and would experience the relaxation of that moment with his family. As Shawn went through the exercise, she massaged Jack's shoulders and upper back, helping him to feel more relaxed and in control of his emotional state.

After several sessions, Jack felt a boost in confidence and made a reservation to fly from Pennsylvania to Chicago, Illinois. Because this was his first flight in months, Shawn went along to help him remember the guided-imagery steps should he panic. The trip was a success. Shawn reminded him several times to calm down and think of the lakeside scene, and Jack responded immediately. When the plane took a sudden dip because of wind currents, Jack felt anxious for a few seconds but then closed his eyes and focused on the visualization exercise. Once he was on the ground in Chicago, Jack was confident that he could conquer his fear of flying and successfully continued his career in sales.

What Is It?

Guided imagery, also called visualization, is a method of communication between body and mind that utilizes perception, position, and movement. It involves imagining relaxing situations—such as a sunset on the beach, a flowing mountain waterfall, or a brilliant mountain sunrise—especially in a stressful situation, using the following thought processes:

+ Vision
+ Smell
+ Taste

- Touch
- Position
- Movement

During imagery, you will make an effort to smell the flowers and trees, sense the breeze or temperature, feel the texture of the surface under your feet, hear all the sounds in nature. While some people are better at imagining than others, anyone can master this simple, inexpensive relaxation technique. You can use guided imagery during massage or other touch therapy to boost relaxation and feelings of serenity and peacefulness. Much like learning to play the piano or tennis, mastering guided imagery involves time, patience, and practice; it is a skill that cannot be rushed.

Where Did It Come From?
Imagery is basic to imagination and linked to many types of faith healing or mind over body. Guided imagery as a healing tool has been used throughout the centuries and is connected to the placebo effect and the power of suggestion. There is evidence that shamanism, a folk method of healing with imagination, occurred thousands of years ago in Asia, then moved to Australia, Europe, and the Americas. Early Greek physicians used imagination and the study of dreams for healing purposes. In the 1920s, imagery was used in medicine to help treat illnesses such as asthma, headaches, and back pain. Later on, imagery was implemented in nursing practices and used with therapeutic touch and other energy-based therapies. Today, guided imagery is used by many popular alternative medicine proponents such as Dean Ornish and Larry Dossey.

How Does It Work?
To practice guided imagery, you need to be alone in a quiet environment without distractions. You may sit in a comfortable chair

or lie down on the floor, couch, or bed. Try to visualize a peaceful, relaxing scene, perhaps a vacation spot you have enjoyed in the mountains or at the seashore. Whatever the scene is, focus on this place. Try to recapture the moment as you imagine its sounds, smells, textures, and feelings. Become more aware of your breathing and anxiety level as you continue your focus, and do not let outside stimuli interrupt.

What's It Good For?

Studies have shown that with guided imagery, you can reduce your anxiety level during stressful times and even lower your heart rate and blood pressure. As you continuously visualize a positive healing image, you may significantly contribute to your own well-being.

If you have trouble imagining scenes and images to destress, listen to sounds of waves or thunderstorms to trigger thoughts of natural settings. Relaxation tapes and CDs with nature sounds can be purchased at any music or department store or on the Internet.

Where's the Science?

In a pilot study at Cedars-Sinai Medical Center, researchers found that acupuncture, massage, and guided imagery eased pain after bypass surgery. In the study, twenty patients were assigned to acupuncture and massage groups after they left the intensive-care unit, typically the day after surgery. The guided-imagery group received therapy before, during, and after surgery. Acupuncture therapy consisted of stimulating points related to relaxation and anxiety as determined by three experienced acupuncturists from the Emperor's College of Traditional Oriental Medicine in California. Some of the patients also received treatment for specific areas of pain. The massage group received therapy for muscles likely to spasm after bypass surgery. A clinical psychologist helped design an audio message that the guided-imagery group listened to. In addition to relaxing the patient, the message explained the procedure that they were undergoing and the origin of some of the pain they might experience. In the exit interview, nineteen of twenty patients in the acupuncture group thought it was very helpful, and similar results were achieved in the other two groups. Some patients described their therapy as "absolutely extraordinary."

MUSIC THERAPY

What Is It?
Music therapy has been proven to be an effective nonpharmacologic approach to assist in reducing fear, anxiety, stress, or grief, no matter what your age.

Composer and researcher Steven Halpern says that certain musical forms can transport the listener's brain into the alpha wave, a state of relaxation much like meditation. Music will allow you to explore personal feelings, make positive changes in mood and emotional states, have a sense of control over life through successful experiences, sort through nagging problems, and resolve inner conflict.

Where Did It Come From?
The effect of this natural tranquilizer on the human spirit can be tied to Pythagoras, the sixth-century B.C. philosopher and mathematician who is considered the founder of music therapy. In the 1940s, veterans' hospitals had volunteers who played music for the wounded solders. The results were so positive that the Veterans Affairs added music-therapy programs.

How Does It Work?
In its simplest form, all you need to incorporate music therapy with any bodywork technique is a tape or CD player with head-

phones, CDs, or tapes. Then choose music that matches your personal needs, moods, and tastes, from New Age "mood" music to rock to classical music.

What's It Good For?

Today there are more than five thousand registered music therapists in the U.S. who use music to soothe—and, some speculate, heal—some physiological and psychological problems. Even surgeons reported performing better when they selected the music played in the operating room. A recent survey of 308 men and women found that exercising and listening to music were the most successful ways for them to get out from under a dark cloud. The *Journal of Personality and Social Psychology* reported that twenty-six psychotherapists rated music and physical activity as smart ways to enhance mood. Children, adolescents, adults, the elderly, those with mental-health needs, developmental and learning disabilities, Alzheimer's disease and other aging-related conditions, substance-abuse problems, brain injuries, physical disabilities, and acute and chronic pain, including mothers in labor, can all benefit.

Many believe that music is as powerful as any medical therapy, since it uniquely accesses the nervous system and brain. In many neurological disorders, such as Alzheimer's, music can help the patient get in touch with something familiar.

Where's the Science?

In a recent study from the University of Wisconsin at Milwaukee, heart-attack survivors in a hospital ward said they felt less anxious immediately after listening to classical music. This change was reflected in their bodies as their heart rates slowed from an average of 79 beats per minute to 71; the average number of breaths they took dropped from 17 to 16 per minute. They also showed an increase in heart-rate variability, a sign that their hearts were growing stronger and more flexible.

When you're under stress, your body releases epinephrine, nor-epinephrine, and other compounds that set your heart racing and increase blood pressure. Researchers in this study believed the music distracted patients from their fears and focused their minds on something more soothing than memories of the heart attack.

Matching creative juices with technical lab studies, composers and researchers are turning out compositions, from classical music to babbling brooks, specifically designed to relax you and reduce mental fatigue and lower stress. In choosing music to destress, try to find arrangements that have one beat per second, many low tones, a lot of strings, and no percussion or brass.

THE FAITH FACTOR

In this health-conscious age, most people seek healers of the mind and spirit, not just mechanics of the body. That's why the use of touch therapies is soaring, as people demand more compassion, more listening, and less lecturing. According to recent polls, two out of three people would like to address spiritual issues with their doctors; half would even like their doctors to pray with them.

Researchers in the field of psychoneuroimmunology (mind/body interplay) report growing evidence on the positive effects of faith in God or a Higher Power on your health. These experts contend that the human body has a powerful sacramental dimension, and those who acknowledge this with a strong sense of higher purpose—a body/soul connectedness—are the ones who are more likely to stay with programs that lead to optimal health. This does not mean that faith in God or a Higher Power should ever replace medical treatment. However, having faith in something greater than yourself offers a type of curative power, helping you to disconnect unhealthy worries and replace them with soothing belief.

In Greek, the word for faith is *pistis*, which means the act of giving one's trust. Trusting in God or a Higher Power permits us to trust and commit to proven medical, nutritional, or fitness regimes we know will benefit us. According to the latest medical research, faith is healthy and even healing. Many studies have found that people who are active in religious organizations and regularly attend group functions report lower blood pressure, less depression, and greater longevity. Perhaps the most famous faith study done on prayer was conducted by Dr. Randolph Byrd, a cardiologist at the University of California at San Francisco Medical Center. He took 393 people who had been admitted to the hospital for heart attack. All of the subjects received the same high-tech, state-of-the-art coronary care, but half were also prayed for by name by prayer groups around the country. No one knew who was being prayed for—the patients, the doctors, the nurses. The prayed-for group experienced fewer deaths and intubations, faster recovery, and didn't use as many potent medications.

PRAYER AND MEDITATION

What Is It?

Prayer and meditation mean different things to different people. Prayer can be used in a religious setting as a heartfelt pleading to God or a Higher Power, or it can be similar to meditation—a cleansing process that allows you to be mindful of the moment without reacting to what you observe, see, or hear. Mindfulness is a moment-to-moment nonjudgmental awareness. At the heart of Buddhist meditation, mindfulness is ultimately about paying attention and cultivating clarity of mind, compassion, and self-love.

Where Did It Come From?

Some forms of prayer and meditation have been practiced for centuries throughout history, whether for physical healing, emotional stability, or to rid the body of evil spirits. As far back as 3,000 years with the Indian yogic practices, cultures have thrived on the spiritual powers within the human existence. Both prayer and meditation were discussed in early Christian and Hebrew literature, as well as in Buddhist writings, where meditation was said to bring about a balance of psychological equilibrium.

How Does It Work?

When you pray or meditate in a mindful state, your brain produces alpha and theta waves consistent with serenity and happiness, allowing your harried thoughts a reprieve. Prayer and meditation can cause a generalized reduction in multiple physiological and biochemical markers, resulting in decreased heart and respiration rate, decreased plasma cortisol (a major stress hormone), decreased pulse rate, and increased EEG (electroencephalogram) activity. Groundbreaking research reveals that these disciplines can also reconfigure the brain biology, triggering therapeutic biochemical and neurological changes. This reconfiguration can make a big difference in one's health and well-being. Just as scientists have found that positive beliefs can engender wellness (the placebo effect), they also have found that negative beliefs and influences can induce illness (the nocebo effect).

What's It Good For?

Meditation or prayer is used effectively alongside massage techniques to minimize the pain and anxiety of labor in childbirth. Meditative techniques are also a key element in the arthritis self-help course at Stanford University. More than a hundred thousand people with arthritis have taken the twelve-hour course and learned meditation-style relaxation exercises as part of a comprehensive self-care program. Graduates report a 15 to 20 percent reduction in pain.

Where's the Science?

In a study published in the *Journal of Holistic Nursing* (December 2000), researchers from the University of Florida and Wayne State University found that most older adults use prayer more than any other alternative health remedy to help manage the stress in their lives. In addition, nurse researchers found that prayer is the most frequently reported alternative treatment used by seniors to feel better or maintain health in general. Ninety-six percent of older adults reported using prayer to cope specifically with stress, and 84 percent reported using prayer more than other alternative remedies to feel better or to maintain their health. Of thirty-two alternative therapies, prayer is used more often than exercise, heat, relaxation techniques, humor, or herbal remedies to maintain overall health.

BIOFEEDBACK

Katrina's Surprising Cure
A Bout with TMJ Ends

After trying various types of mind/body exercises without success, an osteopathic physician referred thirty-six-year-old Katrina Lydel from Pittsburgh, Pennsylvania, to a biofeedback therapist. "I was an introvert and a stuffer, meaning that I kept all emotions stuffed deep inside me. If someone wronged me, rather than confronting the person, I stuffed it inside and never dealt with it. After experiencing a great deal of stress several years ago, the decades of inner turmoil started to manifest in physical symptoms. I was experiencing TMJ from clenching my teeth and jaws at night, and my blood pressure started to increase. My doctor felt I needed to work with a therapist in order to learn how stress was affecting my physical body.

"I learned that the term 'emotion' means outward motion, and how we express our feelings is with our bodies. For example, when most people are angry, they want to lash out with their mouths by yelling or with their arms or shoulder, hitting or pushing the other person away. I was taught 'good girls' never did this, so I always bit my tongue and clenched my fists but hid them so no one could see that I was angry.

"After seeing how I held my tension, the biofeedback therapist explained that when I repressed the expression of emotions, I unconsciously tightened the musculature that should be involved in that expression. That's why I developed TMJ, because I suppressed the very words I should have spoken."

What Is It?

If, after trying some of the mind/body techniques in this chapter, you are still having trouble calming down from daily stress, you may want to look into biofeedback. Biofeedback can allow you to have conscious control over body functions that usually occur automatically—the heartbeat, blood pressure, muscle tension, pain response, and brain waves have all been targeted. Eastern mystics used biofeedback techniques thousands of years ago as they controlled their skin temperature, blood pressure, heart rate, and other involuntary functions through intense concentration.

How Does It Work?

With biofeedback, you are connected to a machine that informs you and your therapist when you are physically tensing and relaxing your body. Through sensors placed over specific muscle sites, the therapist will read the tension in your muscles, heart rate, breathing pattern, the amount of sweat produced, or body temperature. Any one or all of these readings can tell the therapist if you are learning to relax. The ultimate goal of biofeedback is to learn to use this skill for facing the real lions and tigers of life. It can help you control your heart rate, blood pressure, breathing patterns, and muscle tension when you are *not* hooked up to the machine.

Some common types of biofeedback include:

• *Electromyographic (EMG) biofeedback:* This type provides feedback on muscle tension and works well for patients with anxiety disorders or chronic pain.

• *Electrodermal (EDR) biofeedback:* It measures subtle changes in amounts of perspiration.

• *Thermal biofeedback:* The temperature of the skin is measured and is used in teaching hand warming. This has been found to help relieve migraine headaches and can benefit those with Raynaud's disease, which causes the blood vessels in the fingers, toes, ears, and nose to constrict.

• *Finger-pulse biofeedback:* The finger pulse records heart rate and force and is useful for measuring anxiety or cardiovascular symptoms.

• *Respiration feedback:* This type of biofeedback shows the rate, volume, rhythm, and location of each breath.

Where Did It Come From?
Biofeedback derived from various discoveries that all showed humans have an inate ability to control bodily and mental processes.

It was around 1926 when a group of scientists coined the term "biofeedback," meaning biological reactions can be voluntarily influenced by feedback. This term was later adopted in 1969 by a group in Santa Monica, California. At first biofeedback was used strictly by those who were familiar with eastern philosophies. Today, this alternative therapy is popular in clinical settings and has helped many regain control over body functions.

What's It Good For?

Any bodily process that can be measured can be controlled through biofeedback. It is especially effective in relieving chronic pain, particularly tension headaches. However, it can also help relieve temporomandibular joint dysfunction (TMJ), neck and shoulder pain, anxiety, irritable bowel syndrome (IBS), epilepsy, asthma, Raynaud's disease, attention deficit/hyperactivity disorder (ADHD), hypertension, and incontinence; and it can aid in neuromuscular reeducation.

Where's the Science?

One of the most common uses for biofeedback is in pain reduction, specifically, with stress-related pain that is nonspecific. Temporomandibular joint disorder (TMJ) is a painful musculoskeletal condition that is poorly understood but affects many. Researchers have found that psychological approaches including biofeedback, relaxation, and cognitive-behavioral therapy give the best relief for TMJ. New clinical trial data presented in *Current Pain and Headache Reports* (October 2001) showed that a successful approach to treating TMJ involved tailoring psychological and educational treatments, including biofeedback, to the patient's psychosocial profiles.

Credentials

Healthcare professionals must have special training in biofeedback, as well as supervised clinical experience after training. If you are unsure about your therapist's credentials in biofeedback, ask about previous training and the amount of experience.

THAI YOGA MASSAGE AIDS IN HEALING

Yoga is a classical Indian practice that is built on the foundation of ethics (*yama*) and personal discipline (*niyama*). It is used to relieve stress, achieve mind/body connectedness, and heal pain. Thai yoga massage combines the best of yoga and massage, with roots in both the ancient healing traditions of Ayurveda and Thai Buddhism. Instead of going through the various postures, the therapist gives you a full-body massage that combines palming and thumbing along the energy channels and acupoints along the body, along with gentle stretching, movement, and breath work very similar to t'ai chi.

With Thai yoga massage, the therapist uses his or her own hands, arms, elbows, feet, and legs to gently guide the client through yoga postures. This is like a therapeutic dance that helps to boost relaxation and spiritual energy.

Because yoga is a type of mind/body therapy, the postures or movements are structured to stretch the mind and body beyond their normal limits, then make them act in unison again. Using deep breathing, concentration techniques, and body poses, you learn to calm your mind and increase flexibility and strength. *Pranayama*, which is the conscious focus on and control of breath to heal disease, is an important part of yoga.

Thai yoga massage can help relieve mild aches and pains, menstrual cramps, endometriosis, menopausal symptoms, and lower back pain. It can also increase flexibility and coordination, reduce stress, and promote deep relaxation. Breath exercises done with different yoga positions can increase blood circulation.

Yoga relaxes your body, and the various positions can help to improve your breathing, ease constipation, improve skin tone, and increase respiration.

FIND A MIND/BODY THERAPY THAT WORKS

If you still feel too much tension, even after a relaxing massage or bodywork, find the mind/body exercise that best helps you to elicit the relaxation response. All of these therapies are easy to learn and, when combined with a relaxing massage or other therapy, they can help to reduce symptoms of stress.

CHAPTER NINE

Who's Paying the Bill?

"*The* doctor will see you now." How many times have you sat for hours in the doctor's waiting room only to be given a lifestyle prescription of "get more rest," "lose weight," or "exercise more"? For some people, hearing that they are ultimately responsible for self-care is an eye-opener. Yet most of us have become so frustrated with managed care that assuming responsibility for our own health is the most logical decision. After all, there is no magic pill that will ward off stress-related illnesses.

Managed-care organizations (MCOs), such as health-maintenance organizations (HMOs) and preferred-provider organizations (PPOs), have brought drastic changes to the health-care debate. Not only are more than 90 percent of Americans covered by managed care, many policyholders are at the mercy of a gatekeeper, a primary-care physician who dictates what tests or specialists can or cannot be used. While managed care was formulated to provide excellence in health care with lowered costs, it has not exactly turned out that way. In many cases, the care is substandard and the exorbitant cost of treatment is prohibitive. If you need a routine outpatient, minimally invasive surgical procedure, you can figure on spending at least $5,000 to

$6,000. While managed care will pick up some of the tab, you will still incur out-of-pocket costs, and that digs into the already strapped budget of most people.

What's the answer? Should we continue to rely on conventional medical care and the approval of our managed-care system to keep us well, even with its limitations? To some degree, yes—especially for preventive tests, immunizations, and "the big stuff," such as surgery or treatment for cancer and other serious diseases. But many now agree that it's only through responsibility and persistence on your part—not your doctor's—that you can experience optimal health and healing. This is not to say that conventional medicine is to be ignored in any regard. Rather, it should be complemented by the utmost intent to synchronize your mind, body, and spirit. In order to achieve optimal health, you must risk embracing the complex substrate of mysterious life-giving and life-denying spiritual forces, then learn highly effective ways to accept responsibility for self-care. Prevention has become the prime word associated with alternative medicine, but it is ironic how few people are willing to pay the price to stay well and out of the doctor's office. Considering that Americans make about 1.5 billion office visits to doctors every year for such preventable problems as colds, hypertension, migraines, backaches, gastrointestinal complaints, unexplained fatigue, and obesity, the annual cost of staying well is a mere pittance compared with the annual cost of getting well.

THE ANNUAL COST OF STAYING WELL	THE ANNUAL COST OF GETTING WELL
Daily walking free	Coronary bypass surgery $40,000+
Electrocardiogram $80	Hospitalization for heart attack $18,200
Quitting cigarettes free	Lung-cancer treatment $34,000+

PSA test $75	Prostate-cancer surgery $21,000+
Yearly mammogram $130	Breast cancer/mastectomy $7,500+
Preventive dental care $175	Gum-disease surgery $1,500+
Sunscreen $126	Skin-cancer treatment $6,000+
Bone-density scan $125	Hospitalization for broken hip $16,871
Massage/bodywork $40	Medication for hypertension $1,300
Social support free	Weekly psychotherapy $5,400+
Mind/body exercises free	Prozac (or other meds) $500+

Perhaps the facts speak for themselves. If you want to stay healthy for the rest of your life, it is cheaper (and wiser) to make prevention a priority than to risk disrupting your body's healing system. Alternative medicine may be the welcome light at the end of the long, dark tunnel.

Four out of ten adults in the U.S. (42 percent) have used some type of complementary treatment this past year; holistic health coverage is in great demand. The total number of visits to alternative-medicine providers increased from 427 million in 1990 to 629 million in 1997—an increase of 47 percent—while the number of visits to all primary-care physicians declined over the same period. According to a survey conducted by Landmark Healthcare and InterActive Solutions, access to alternative medicine was a key factor for two thirds of Americans in choosing a health plan. Oxford Health Plans was the first major health-care program in the United States to offer a network of credentialed alternative-medicine providers, each held to strict certification and experience standards. Oxford members now have access to more than twenty-two hundred alternative-medicine providers, all of whom are recredentialed every two years. They include:

- Nutritionists
- Massage therapists
- Acupuncturists
- Chiropractors
- Naturopaths
- Yoga instructors

Even though some health plans provide alternative therapies, on the whole, the United States lags behind other countries in supporting holistic health treatments. In Germany, massage therapy is covered by national health insurance. In China, it is fully integrated into the health-care system: The hospitals have massage wards. In one Shanghai hospital, the massage department covers two floors. In this country, the medical use of massage began to diminish in the early part of this century with the evolution of pharmaceutical, surgical, and technological medicine. It reached its lowest point from the 1930s through the '50s because it was considered too time-intensive for the modern physician. Massage-therapy duties were gradually handed over to nurses, who eventually became the physical therapists of the modern era.

Boomers Seek Massage

In years past, those who sought alternative therapies were thought of as uneducated or gullible. Today's studies reveal that it is the educated, middle- or upper-middle-class consumer who is most health-conscious and who is seeking full participation in self-care with alternative therapies.

It may surprise you that of all the age groups, those most likely to seek massage are the baby boomers, according to a survey taken by Oxford Health Plans. When offered, 100 percent of workers age 45 to 54 took advantage of a massage, while only 60 percent of those age 18 to 34, 20 percent of those age 35 to 44, and 50 percent of those age 55 and older did.

Unconventional Therapies Move to Mainstream

Although there is some feeling among the most conventional health-care professionals that alternative therapies need to stay away from mainstream medicine, many renowned medical schools are delving into all types of unconventional therapies. Not wanting to limit healing modalities, 75 of the 125 medical schools in the U.S. (60 percent) offer courses in alternative medicine. At Duke University's Department of Psychiatry, herbal medicine has been added to its large research program, with a $4.3 million grant to study St.-John's-wort. The Center for Aging at Duke receives significant funding to study the effects of spirituality and religion on health. In related clinical research, the Durham Veterans Affairs Medical Center is sponsoring the Monitoring and Actualization of Noetic Training (MANTRA) project where patients undergoing cardiac catheterization are randomized to a control group or one of four complementary therapies, including meditation, imagery, healing touch, or remote prayer by several off-site prayer groups from around the world. Other well-known medical schools, such as Harvard and Stanford, are also integrating alternative therapies into their conventional-medicine curriculum.

In the United States, Congress formed the National Center for Complementary and Alternative Medicine as part of the National Institutes of Health to help evaluate alternative medical treatments and determine their effectiveness. Over time, this organization will establish safe guidelines to help people choose appropriate alternative and complementary therapies.

HOW TO UNDERSTAND YOUR POLICY

To see if massage and other touch therapies are covered in your managed-care plan, you have to be a savvy consumer. This takes some homework: Study your policy, investigate the extras provided to you, ask pertinent questions ahead of time, and even push your provider to pay if the therapy seems reasonable and works in your case. While you can always pay for alternative therapies, it's more cost-efficient to get your health plan to cover them.

Your managed-care contract is a mechanism to obtain both conventional and alternative health care. When you sign the contract, you agree to its specific terms, such as choosing a physician from a panel of health-care providers, referral to specialists or for specialized testing, and choices in alternative therapies, if any.

Ask for and carefully read your managed-care plan's written policy, a certificate of coverage. This material should be easy to understand, as well as detailed and comprehensive, giving the exact parameters of your policy. If you have questions, call your plan representative. If your plan is through your employer, talk to the human-resources manager. Never assume that any service will be covered—be sure it will! Ask questions ahead of time.

To see if any alternative treatments, such as massage, are covered in your plan, go through the plan line by line to look for:

- Alternative medical care
- Preventive care
- Hospital of choice
- Prescription drugs
- Homeopathic remedies
- Herbal remedies
- Worldwide coverage
- Major medical coverage
- X-ray/lab tests
- Maternity/reproductive/midwifery
- Mental-health services
- Hospital services
- Specific alternative therapies
  Acupuncture, Ayurvedic medicine, Biofeedback, Birthing centers and midwives, Bodywork and therapeutic massage, Chelation therapy, Chinese

medicine, Chiropractic, Detoxification, Environmental medicine, Herbal therapy, Homeopathy, Hydrotherapy, Light-box therapy, Magnet therapy, Mind/body treatments, Naturopathy, Nutritional supplements, Nutritional therapy, Osteopathy

Getting Through the Gate

Managed-care organizations, particularly HMOs, typically require patients to obtain referrals from primary-care physicians (known commonly as gatekeepers) to specialists. Some plans may consider alternative-health practitioners specialists and require referrals by the patient's physician. Under these plans, the MCO would not have to pay for the service without a valid referral. Most plans covering alternative medicine have opted to use a fee-for-service payment method that does not require a referral.

Whether from insurance or their own pocket, consumers now spend $2 to $4 billion annually for massages. Since many can't afford the average $45-per-hour fee, insurance policies often determine who gets the therapy and who doesn't. Some states are even considering legislation that would require insurance companies to cover treatments by licensed massage therapists.

Legally Speaking

As public support for alternative medicine grows, managed-care organizations, insurers, and other third-party payers are confronted with legal issues regarding coverage, costs, and payments. For the most part, an MCO or insurer's obligation to provide and pay for alternative-medicine coverage; a plan member's right to alternative medicine for covered services; and a provider's right to receive payment for alternative medicine is based on the contractual obligations. These are contained in the managed-care plan or insurance policy; the alternative-medicine provider's participating-provider agreement, in the case of a managed-care plan; or the patient's insurance policy, in the case of insurance. Many MCOs or insurers specifically exclude coverage for "experimental" or "investigational" treatments, or in the alternative, adopt the Medicare treatment of such services or treatments.

What's Experimental, What's Not?

Most alternative medicine is difficult to measure for effectiveness due to its subjectivity. Remedial success is often dependent upon patient participation, since traditional research protocols, such as laboratory tests and scientific data, are not appropriate for measuring the effectiveness of alternative therapies. As a result, alternative medicine is often classified as experimental or investigational by insurers. Subsequently, the managed-care industry is struggling with the question: When is an alternative-medicine therapy no longer considered experimental?

For many MCOs, the answer to this question determines if the therapy will be covered or excluded. If the treatment has withstood clinical trials showing that it is safe and cost-effective, it should no longer be considered experimental or investigational. Still, these terms are not exact. Because the term "experimental" has many meanings, classification often appears to be more of a financial than a scientific decision. Under some plans and policies, massage or chiropractic is still considered experimental and coverage is denied, even though both modalities have scientific studies to back them up. Yet any plan or policy may classify an alternative medicine as experimental and deny coverage.

There is little consistency among managed-care organizations in determining which treatments are experimental and excluded from coverage. What is deemed experimental by one plan may be standard to another. Therefore, many insurers look to Medicare to design their coverage.

Medicare bases its coverage amounts on whether or not the services are "reasonable and necessary," which means services that are "safe, effective, appropriate, and not experimental." This may include massage, bodywork, and other alternative treatments. Some private insurers have developed an objective process for determining whether a technology is no longer to be considered experimental. Guidelines specify that:

+ The technology must have final approval from the appropriate government regulatory bodies
+ Scientific evidence allows conclusions related to alternative medicine's effect on health
+ The alternative-medicine therapy must improve health outcomes
+ These improvements must be achievable outside the research setting

While most health plans and insurers have relied on scientific or medical research to determine whether an alternative-medicine therapy will be covered, an increasing number now require approval from a medical association and/or an independent board of physicians to provide coverage for an experimental treatment. This may be where the snags occur; how many conventional doctors want to see their patients receive treatment elsewhere, especially from a practitioner who did not "pay their dues" with years of medical school training?

In short, exclusionary clauses in contracts—which preclude coverage of experimental or investigational treatments—are one way insurers can deny coverage for what they consider expensive treatments. The drafting of excluded benefits is a legal challenge to MCO lawyers.

Denying Coverage

In the midst of insurance companies telling you what they will or won't pay, there are still some checks and balances that put the final decision back in your court. Denial of coverage can expose the health-care organization to antitrust, contract, and tort liability. Antitrust issues prohibit two or more health plans from a course of conduct that may constitute a boycott of a particular therapy or treatment. For example, MCO "A" and MCO "B" may not legally agree to exclude massage from coverage. Such conduct could constitute an illegal boycott, or restraint on trade. MCOs must be very careful with the process used for determination of excluded services. Even the hint of impropriety can lead to antitrust liability.

This does not mean that health plans cannot share scientific research. Health plans have a legitimate right to make informed decisions regarding coverage of services. Legal problems arise when documentation and correspondence fail to reflect accurately how they reached the decision.

Contract Concerns

Contract issues focus primarily on the clarity of the language of the insurance policy or managed-care plan. The policy or plan is a contract between the policyholder and the insurance company or MCO. The policyholder agrees to pay the required premiums, and the insurance company agrees to reimburse health-care costs listed in the contract. Litigation usually focuses on any words in the policy that could be interpreted in more than one way. Courts will look to the specific language of the policy in resolving conflicts. If the exclusionary clause is ambiguous, the policyholder may prevail. If it is clear, the court determines whether it can be construed to exclude an alternative-medicine therapy as experimental. In many cases involving ambiguous language in contracts, courts have ruled in favor of coverage because the insurer or MCO wrote the contract provisions. Case law regarding nonreimbursement issues has been inconsistent mainly because the language in managed-care contracts varies significantly among companies.

An important point: Courts will generally require insurers to provide coverage when the contract fails to define experimental treatment or bases the exclusion on unspecified criteria. Some courts have upheld exclusions if the insurer can prove that the treatment is experimental or not medically necessary. Due to the increase in litigation, many HMOs are developing specific guidelines for determining whether a procedure will be covered and are using clear, specific language in the exclusionary clauses.

Questioning Your Coverage

After you read your policy and assess the alternative therapies covered, write down any questions—no matter how trite they may seem—to ask your provider. For example, while your policy may cover massage or bodywork therapies, it may list coverage only for "fibromyalgia, chronic headaches, and back pain." This means that if you are seeking massage or bodywork for stress reduction or neck pain, you will not be reimbursed. Still, if you are in a car accident or have a job-related injury covered by worker's compensation, insurance may cover massage or bodywork prescribed by a physician. If your insurance covers chiropractic or osteopathic, the services of a massage/bodywork practitioner may be covered when prescribed by a chiropractor or osteopath.

While you are reading your policy, find out how much is paid for a particular treatment, what the standard deductible is, and if this treatment must have a referral through your gatekeeper. Many HMOs will not touch a treatment unless your primary-care doctor has referred you and the specialist you are referred to is listed on the plan. Sometimes insurers will pay only a portion of the bill for alternative therapies, such as 50 percent, if any at all.

It is important to know that alternative medicine is big business. Billions of dollars are spent out of pocket on alternative therapies annually, and money can talk. Continue up the chain of authority with your insurance company, until you are satisfied that you have spoken with someone who understands your policy. If you still feel you have a case to seek payment, document it and go to small claims court.

To avoid headaches and hassles regarding payment for services, check it out before you need the therapy to ensure the greatest success in using alternative medicine.

Managed Care 101

Managed-Care Term		Your Rights
Health-maintenance organization	(HMO)	Select primary-care physician who refers you to specialists
Preferred-provider organization	(PPO)	Select primary-care physician from a panel of specialists, but no referral needed to see a specialist
Out of Network		Similar to fee-for-service: The physician is not in your insurance plan. Your plan may pay part of the physician's fee, and you are responsible for the difference. If your out-of-network physician recommends a test and the primary-care physician does not agree, you may have to pay for the test.

TALKING TO YOUR DOCTOR ABOUT ALTERNATIVE THERAPIES

At this time, many managed-care providers acknowledge the benefits of massage and other alternative therapies for prevention and treatment of disease. This is particularly true in the twenty-five states and the District of Columbia where massage therapists are licensed by state regulatory bodies. If massage therapists are not licensed in your state, therapeutic massage may still be covered or reimbursable. Due to public demand, competition for market share, and perceived cost savings, MCOs are becoming more open to alternative-medicine therapies.

Investigate the Practitioner and the Therapy

Perhaps you've been thinking about trying massage or another form of touch therapy to relieve stress, or acupuncture for chronic pain. Or maybe you've already been to a massage therapist and you want to talk to your doctor about its effect on your overall health. It's important to interview the therapist ahead of time to make sure this is the right professional to serve you. Review the background and professional credentials of your chosen practitioner. Ask specific questions about the services you will be receiving. Some questions to ask include:

- What are your credentials? Are you licensed?
- Where did you do your training? How many hours did you study?
- Do you have any clients I could ask for references?
- What will the treatment involve?
- How long will I need the treatment?
- What are the advantages and disadvantages of this therapy as opposed to others? Can I use the treatment along with conventional medicine?
- Is this treatment safe? Are there studies to support it?
- How much will each session cost? Does insurance cover the cost?
- When should I see results?
- Are there any dangerous side effects I should be aware of?
- Can my doctor call you regarding the treatment to keep communication open?

TOUCH LETS EVERYONE CELEBRATE OPTIMAL HEALTH

As you take advantage of the information in *Miracle Touch* and follow the various touch therapies and relaxation techniques, you will be well on your way to enjoying optimal health—mentally, physically, emotionally, and spiritually. No matter what your health situation, there are healing therapies that can help to ease your symptoms, reverse or even resolve illness, and let you experience a greater quality of life—all your life!

Notes

1: Touch: Help, Hype, or Hoax?
p. 18 Drummond, Tammerlin. *Touch Early and Often. Time.com.* Health Vol. 152, No. 4. (July 27, 1998)
http://www.time.com/time/magazine/1998/dom/980727/health.touch_early_and_o14.html.

p. 19 Davis, Phyllis, *The Power of Touch* (Carlsbad, CA: Hay House, 1999), p. 83.

p. 20 Fields, T., "American Adolescents Touch Each Other Less and Are More Aggressive Toward Their Peers As Compared with French Adolescents," *Adolescence,* Vol. 34, No. 136 (Winter 1999), pp. 753–58.

p. 22 Collinge, William, Ph.D., *Subtle Energy: Awakening to the Unseen Forces in Our Lives* (New York: Warner Books, 1998).

2: Steeped in Ancient Traditions
p. 40 Oschmann, James L., Ph.D., *Readings of the Scientific Basis of Bodywork: The Natural Science of Healing* (Dover, NH: Nature's Own Research Association, 1977), p. 82.

p. 47 Fosshage, James L., "The Meanings of Touch in Psychoanalysis: A Time for Reassessment" (http://www.psychoanalyticinquiry.com/vol20no1.html).

3: From Magnets to Manual Manipulation
p. 74 Palmer, D. D., *Textbook of the Science, Art and Philosophy of Chiropractic* (Portland, OR: Portland Printing, 1910), p. 111.

p. 77 Kragthorpe, Kurt. *Showdown Notes: Back Injury Delayed; Tewell's Senior Debut.* The Salt Lake Tribune (August 21, 2000), p. C3.

4: *Bodywork, Massage, and New Age Trends*
p. 87 Benor, Daniel J., M.D., "Intuitive Diagnosis," *Subtle Energies and Energy Medicine Journal*, Vol. 3, No. 2 (1992), pp. 41–64.

5: *The Mystery of Faith Healing*
p. 124 LeShan, Lawrence, *The Medium, the Mystic and the Physicist* (New York: Penguin, 1995), p. 93.

6: *Centering on Therapeutic Touch*
p. 144 Benor, Daniel J., M.D., 1994. Reprinted with permission of the author.

References

Agarwal, K.N., A. Gupta, R. Pushkarna, et al., "Effects of Massage and Use of Oil on Growth, Blood Flow and Sleep Pattern in Infants," *Indian Journal of Medical Research*, Vol. 112 (December 2000), pp. 212–17.

Andersson, G.B., T. Lucente, A.M. Davis, et al., "A Comparison of Osteopathic Spinal Manipulation with Standard Care for Patients with Low Back Pain," *New England Journal of Medicine*, Vol. 341, No. 19 (November 1999), pp. 1426–31.

Avants, S.K., et al., "A Randomized Controlled Trial of Auricular Acupuncture for Cocaine Dependence," *Archives of Internal Medicine*, Vol. 160, No. 15 (August 2000), pp. 2305–12.

Ballegaard, S., S. Norrelund, D.F. Smith, "Cost-Benefit of Combined Use of Acupuncture, Shiatsu and Lifestyle Adjustment for Treatment of Patients with Severe Angina Pectoris," *Acupuncture and Electrotherapy Research*, Vol. 21, Nos. 3–4 (July–December 1996), pp. 187–97.

Benford, M.S., J. Talnagi, D.B. Doss, et al., "Gamma Radiation Fluctuations during Alternative Healing Therapy," *Alternative Therapies in Health and Medicine* Vol. 5, No. 4 (July 1999), pp. 51–56.

Benson, H., and M. Stark, "Reason to Believe," *Natural Health* (May–June 1996), p. 74.

Benson, H., et al., *The Wellness Book: The Comprehensive Guide to Maintaining Health and Treating Stress-Related Illness* (New York: Birch Lane Press, 1992).

Benson, H., et al., "The Placebo Effect: a Neglected Asset in the Care of Patients," *Journal of the American Medical Association*, Vol. 232 (1975), pp. 1225–27.

Benson, H., et al., "Relaxation Response: Bridge Between Psychiatry and Medicine," *Medical Clinics of North America*, Vol. 61 (1977), pp. 929–38.

Borysenko, J., *Minding the Body, Mending the Mind*. (New York: Bantam, 1987).

Bowman, Jo, "TV Healer Prepares to Work 'Miracles' in SAR," *South China Morning Post* (May 9, 2001).

Diego, M.A., N.A. Jones, T. Fields, et al., "Aromatherapy Positively Affects Mood, EEG Patterns of Alertness and Math Computations," *International Journal of Neuroscience*, Vol. 96, Nos. 3–4 (December 1998), pp. 217–24.

Dossey, L., *Healing Words* (New York: HarperCollins, 1993).

Dossey, L., *Meaning and Medicine* (New York: Bantam, 1991).

Dunn, K.S., A.L. Horgas, "The Prevalence of Prayer as a Spiritual Self-care Modality in Elders," *Journal of Holistic Nursing*, Vol. 18, No. 4 (December 2000), pp. 337–51.

Elkayam, O., S. Ben Itzhak, E. Avrahami, et al., "Multidisciplinary Approach to Chronic Back Pain: Prognostic Elements of the Outcome," *Clinical and Experimental Rheumatology*, Vol. 14, No. 3 (May–June 1996), pp. 281–88.

Fakouri, C., P. Jones, "Relaxation Rx: Slow-Stroke Back Rub," *Journal of Gerontological Nursing*, Vol. 13 (February 1987), pp. 32–35.

Fawzy, F. I., N. Cousins, N.W. Fawzy, et al., "A Structured Psychiatric Intervention for Cancer Patients. I. Changes Over Time in Methods of Coping and Affective Disturbance," *Archives of General Psychiatry*, Vol. 47, No. 8 (August 1990), pp. 720–25.

Fields, T. "American Adolescents Touch Each Other Less and Are More Aggressive Toward Their Peers as Compared with French Adolescents." *Adolescence*, Vol. 34, No. 136 (Winter 1999), pp. 753–58.

Fields, T., *Touch in Early Development* (New Jersey: Lawrence Erlbaum Associates, 1995).

Fields, T., C. Morrow, C. Valdeon, et al., "Massage Reduces Anxiety in Child and Adolescent Psychiatric Patients," *Journal of the American Academy of Child and Adolescent Psychiatry*, Vol. 31 (1992), pp. 125–31.

Fields, T., G. Ironson, F. Scafidi, et al., "Massage Therapy Reduces Anxiety and Enhances EEG Pattern of Alertness and Math Computations," *International Journal of Neuroscience*, Vol. 86, Nos. 3–4 (September 1996), pp. 197–205.

Fields, T., S. Schanberg, F. Scafidi, et al., "Tactile/Kinesthetic Stimulation Effects on Preterm Neonates," *Pediatrics*, Vol. 77 (May 1986), pp. 654–58.

Fiske, J. C. Dickinson, "The Role of Acupuncture in Controlling the Gagging Reflex Using a Review of Ten Cases," *British Dental Journal*, Vol. 190, No. 11 (June 2001), pp. 611–13.

Foltz-Gray, D., "My Happiness Gene," *Health* (September 1997), pp. 60–62.

Gallup, G., Jr., *Religion in America 1990* (Princeton, N.J.: Princeton Religion Research Center, 1990).

Gerber, R., "Exploring Human Potential," Innerself at http://www.innerself.com.

Goleman, D.J., *The Varieties of the Meditative Experience* (New York: Irvington Publishers, 1977).

Goleman, D.J., *Mind Body Medicine* (New York: Consumer Reports, 1993).

Hadden, J.K., et al., "The Sermon from the Satellite," *Prime Time Preachers*, http://religiousbroadcasting.lib.virginia.edu/primetime/C5.html.

Hafen, B. O., et al., *Health Effects of Attitudes, Emotions and Relationships* (Provo, UT: EMS Associates, 1992).

Hall, N., ed. *Mind/Body Interactions and Disease and Psychoneuroimmunological Aspects of Health and Disease* (Orlando, FL: Health Dateline Press, 1996).

Hardy, M., et al., "Replacement of Drug Therapy for Insomnia by Ambient Odor." *Lancet*, Vol. 346 (1995), p. 701.

House, J. S., et al., "Social Relationships and Health," *Science*, Vol. 241 (July 1988), p. 540.

Irnich, D., N. Behrens, H. Molzen, et al., "Randomised Trial of Acupuncture Compared with Conventional Massage and "Sham" Laser Acupuncture for

Treatment of Chronic Neck Pain," *British Medical Journal*, Vol. 322, No. 7302 (June 2001), pp. 1574–78.

Ironson, G., et al.,"Massage Therapy Is Associated with Enhancement of the Immune System's Cytotoxic Capacity," *International Journal of Neuroscience*, Vol. 84, Nos. 1–4 (February 1996), pp. 205–17.

Kaarda, B., O. Tosteinbo, "Increase of Plasma Beta-Endorphins in Connective Tissue Massage," *General Pharmacology*, Vol. 20 (1989), pp. 487–89.

Katz, J., A. Wowk, D. Culp, et al.,"Pain and Tension Are Reduced Among Hospital Nurses after On-Site Massage Treatments: A Pilot Study," *Journal Perianesthesia Nursing*, Vol. 14, No. 3 (June 1999), pp. 128–33.

Keville, K., M. Green, *Aromatherapy: A Complete Guide to the Healing Art* (Santa Cruse, CA: Crossing Press, 1995).

Krieger, D.,"Healing by the Laying on of Hands as a Facilitator of Bio-energetic Change: the Response of In-vivo Human Hemaglobin," *International Journal of Psychoenergy Systems*, Vol. 1, No. 1 (1976), pp. 121–29.

Krieger, D., *The Therapeutic Touch: How to Use Your Hands to Help or Heal* (Eaglewood Cliffs, NJ: Prentice-Hall, 1979).

Krieger, D., *"Therapeutic Touch and Healing Energies from the Laying on of Hands,"* *Journal of Holistic Health*, Vol. 1 (1975), pp. 23–30.

Krieger, D.,"The Imprimatur of Nursing," *American Journal of Nursing*, Vol. 75 (1975), pp. 784–87.

Krieger, D.,"The Relationship of Touch with Intent to Help or to Heal, to Subjects In-vivo Hemoglobin Values," *Proceedings of the Ninth American Nurses Association Research Conference* (New York: American Nurses Association, 1973), pp. 39–59.

Krieger, D.,"Therapeutic Touch: Searching for Evidence of Physiological Change," *American Journal of Nursing*, Vol. 79, No. 4 (1979), pp. 660–62.

Laumer, U., M. Bauer, M. Fichter, et al.,"Therapeutic Effects of the Feldenkrais Method 'Awareness Through Movement' in Patients with Eating Disorders," *Psychotherapy and Psychosomatic Medical Psychology*, Vol. 47, No. 5 (May 1997), pp. 170–80.

LeShan, L.L., *You Can Fight for Your Life: Emotional Factors in the Causation of Cancer* (New York: M. Evans, 1977).

Levin, J. S. "Religion and Health: Is There an Association, Is It Valid, and Is It Casual?", *Social Science and Medicine*, Vol. 38 (June 1994), pp. 1475–82.

McKechnie, A., F. Wilson, N. Watson, et al., "Anxiety States: A Preliminary Report on the Value of Connective Tissue Massage," *Journal of Psychosomatic Research*, Vol. 27, No. 2 (1983), pp. 125–29.

Miller, C., "Mental Powers: Divine Power over Blood Pressure," *Longevity* (September 1989), p. 78.

Modica, P., "The Ancient Art of Acupuncture Gets FDA Approval," *Medical Tribune News Service* (May 24, 1996).

Moore, T., Care of the Soul: A Guide for Cultivating Depth and Sacredness in Everyday Life (New York: HarperCollins, 1992), pp. 59–118.

Mustafa, T. K.C. Srivastava, "Ginger (Zingiber officinale) in Migraine Headache," *Journal of Ethnopharmacology*, Vol. 29, No. 3 (July 1990), pp. 267–73.

Nicolson, N., C. Storms, R. Ponds, et al., "Salivary Cortisol Levels and Stress Reactivity in Human Aging," *Journals of Gerontology. Series A, Biological Sciences and Medical Sciences*, Vol. 52, No. 2 (March 1997), pp. M68–75.

National Institutes of Health, "Alternative Medicine, Expanding Medical Horizons: A Report to the National Institutes of Health on Alternative Medical Systems and Practices in the United States," NIH Publication, No. 94-066 (1994).

Olson, K., J. Hanson, "Using Reiki to Manage Pain: A Preliminary Report," *Cancer Prevention and Control*, Vol. 1, No. 2 (June 1997), pp. 108–13.

Olson, M., N. Sneed, M. La Via, et al., "Stress-Induced Immunosuppression and Therapeutic Touch," *Alternative Therapies in Health and Medicine*, Vol. 3, No. 2 (March 1997), pp. 68–74.

Ramirez, M. " 'Amma' Brings Message of Love," *Seattle Times* (May 30, 2001).

Reston, J., *New York Times* (July 26, 1971), pp. 1,6.

Sellar, W., et al., *Frankincense & Myrrh: Through the Ages and a Complete Guide to Their Use in Herbalism and Aromatherapy Today* (Woodstock, NY: Beekman Publishing, Inc., 1997).

Sherman, J.J., et al., "Nonpharmacologic Approaches to the Management of Myofascial Temporomandibular Disorders," *Current Pain and Headache Report*, Vol. 5, No. 5 (October 2001), pp. 421–31.

State of Wisconsin v. S.R. Jansheski, tried in the District Court of Milwaukee, WI., December 1910. Portions of testimony reprinted in *A Chiropractic Catechism* (American Medical Association Bureau of Legal Medicine and Legislation), p. 6.

Sung, B.H., *American Journal of Hypertension*, Vol. 13 (2000), pp. 185A–186A.

Suomi, S.J. "Social Rehabilitation of Isolate-reared Monkeys," *Developmental Psychology*, Vol. 6 (1972), pp. 487–96.

Tuchin, P.J., et al., "A Randomized Controlled Trial of Chiropractic Spinal Manipulative Therapy for Migraine," *Journal of Manipulative and Physiological Therapeutics*, Vol. 23, No. 2 (February 2000), pp. 91–95.

Turner, J.G., et al., "The Effect of Therapeutic Touch on Pain and Anxiety in Burn Patients," *Journal of Advanced Nursing*, Vol. 28, No. 1 (July 1998), pp. 10–20.

Turner, R.A., et al., "Preliminary Research on Plasma Oxytocin in Normal Cycling Women: Investigating Emotion and Interpersonal Distress," *Psychiatry*, Vol. 62, No. 2 (Summer 1999), pp. 97–113.

Uchino, B. N., et al., "The Relationship Between Social Support and Physiological Processes: A Review with Emphasis on Underlying Mechanisms and Implications for Health," *Psychological Bulletin*, Vol. 119, No. 3 (May 1996), pp. 488–531.

Walton-Hadlock, J. "Primary Parkinson's Disease: The Use of Tuina and Acupuncture in Accord with an Evolving Hypothesis of Its Cause from the Perspective of Chinese Traditional Medicine—Part 2," *American Journal of Acupuncture*, Vol. 27, Nos. 1–2 (1999), pp. 31–49.

Wardell, D.W., J. Engebretson, "Biological Correlates of Reiki Touch Healing," *Journal of Advanced Nursing*, Vol. 33, No. 4 (February 2001), pp. 439–45.

Warner, W.E., *The Woman Evangelist: The Life and Times of Charismatic Evangelist Maria B. Woodworth-Etter* (Metuchen, NJ: The Scarecrow Press, Inc., 1986), pp. 180, 234.

Weintraub, M., "Alternative Medical Care: Shiatsu, Swedish Muscle Massage, and Trigger Point Suppression in Spinal Pain Syndrome," *American Journal of Pain Management*, Vol. 2, No. 2 (1992), pp. 74–78.

Weintraub, M., "Shiatsu, Swedish Muscle Massage, and Trigger Point Suppression in Spinal Pain Syndrome," *American Massage Therapy Journal*, Vol. 31, No. 3 (1992), pp. 99–109.

Winstead-Fry, P., "An Integrative Review and Meta-analysis of Therapeutic Touch Research," *Alternative Therapies and Health Medicine*, Vol. 5 (1999), pp. 58–67.

Wolf, B., "20 Million Hugs: Indian Holy Woman on 'Hugging Tour' of United States and World," *ABC News* (July 15, 2001).

Wright, S.M., "The Use of Therapeutic Touch in the Management of Pain," *Nursing Clinics of North America*, Vol. 22, No. 3 (1987), pp. 705–14.

WEBSITES

Acupressure and Shiatsu: http://www.acupressure.com/

Alternative Health Benefits Service: http://www.alternativeinsurance.com/

American Academy of Medical Acupuncture:
http://www.medicalacupuncture.org/

Amma Center of New Mexico:
http://www.ammacenter.org/pages/about.html

Ammachi.org: The Official Ammachi website: http://www.ammachi.org/

Aston-Patterning: http://www.aston-patterning.com/

Bach Flower Essences: http://www.holisticmed.com/www/bach.html

Benny Hinn Ministries: http://www.bennyhinn.org/index1.cfm

Chiropractic (American Chiropractic Association):
http://www.amerchiro.org/

Ernest Angley Ministries:
http://www.ernestangley.org/Tracts/HTMLs/initial%20evidence.htm

Faith Healing: *The Columbia Encyclopedia*, Sixth Edition, 2001: www.bartleby.com

Global Reiki Network: http://www.reiki.org/

Hellerwork Forum: http://www.alt-med-ed.com/practices/hellerwork.htm

History of Osteopathic Medicine: http://history.aoa-net.org/Osteopathy/timeline.htm

International Chiropractic Association: http://www.chiropractic.org

Kenneth Copeland Ministries: http://www.kcm.org/

Myofascial Release: http://www.myofascial-release.com/

Nurse Healers Professional Associates International: http://www.therapeutic-touch.org/content/ttouch.asp.

Osteopathy: http://www.healthandage.com/html/res/com/ConsModalities/Osteopathycm.html

Osteopathic PreMed FAQ: http://www.studentdoctor.com/do/premedfaq.html

Reflexology: http://www.reflexology.org/

Rosen Method Bodywork and Movement: http://www.rosenmethod.org/

Rupert Sheldrake Interview: http://www.sheldrake.org/

The American Massage Therapy Institute: http://www.amtamassage.org/

The Ayurvedic Institute: http://www.ayurveda.com/

The Chiropractic Resource Organization: http://www.chiro.org

The Complete Guide to the Alexander Technique: http://www.alexandertechnique.com/

The Feldenkrais Method®: http://www.feldenkrais.com/

The Rolf Institute: http://www.rolf.org/

The Trager® Approach: http://www.trager.com/

Index